ELMWOOD PARK PUBLIC LIBRARY
4 CONTI PARKWAY
ELMWOOD PARK, IL 60707
(708) 453-7645/8236

1. A fine is charged for each day a book is kept
   beyond the due date. The Library Board may take
   legal action if books are not returned within three
   months.

2. Books damaged beyond reasonable wear shall be
   paid for.

3. Each borrower is responsible for all books
   charged on this card and for all fines accruing on
   the same.

How to Meet the Right Woman

How to Meet
the Right Woman
A Five-Step Strategy That Really Works

**Roger Ratcliff, David Conaway,
and Diana Ohlsson**

A Citadel Press Book
Published by Carol Publishing Group

Carol Publishing Group Edition, 1998

Copyright © 1996 Roger Ratcliff and David Conaway
All rights reserved. No part of this book may be reproduced in any
form, except by a newspaper or magazine reviewer who wishes to
quote brief passages in connection with a review.

A Citadel Press Book
Published by Carol Publishing Group
Citadel Press is a registered trademark of Carol Communications, Inc.

Editorial, sales and distribution, and rights and permissions
inquiries should be addressed to Carol Publishing Group,
120 Enterprise Avenue, Secaucus, N.J. 07094

In Canada: Canadian Manda Group, One Atlantic Avenue, Suite 105,
Toronto, Ontario M6K 3E7

Carol Publishing Group books may be purchased in bulk at special
discounts for sales promotion, fund-raising, or educational
purposes. Special editions can be created to specifications. For
details, contact Special Sales Department, Carol Publishing Group,
120 Enterprise Avenue, Secaucus, N.J. 07094

Manufactured in the United States of America
10 9 8 7 6 5 4 3 2 1

Library of Congress Cataloging-in-Publication Data
Ratcliff, Roger.
    How to meet the right woman : a five-step strategy that really
works / Roger Ratcliff, David Conaway, and Diana Ohlsson.
        p.   cm.
    "A Citadel Press book."
    ISBN 0-8065-2021-3 (pbk.)
    1. Mate selection   2. Man-woman relationships.   3. Dating (Social
customs)   I. Conaway, David.   II. Ohlsson, Diana.   III. Title.
HQ801.R2583   1996
646.7'7—dc20   96-33580
                                                        CIP

Contents

❦Introduction❦
We Learned the Hard Way

DAVE'S STORY

You may know what it feels like to have a date canceled at the last minute. That happened to me the last time I was on a campaign to find a woman to share my life. I had been looking forward to a date with a woman I had met a few days earlier, but an hour before I was supposed to pick her up she called and said, "I'm going to have to break our date. I put too many activities on my social calendar this week. Tonight I want to stay home."

I hate broken dates, but I didn't sit around feeling depressed. I knew what I had to do and immediately swung into action. Within one hour of her call, I had gone out, then met and made a date with another woman whom I found equally attractive. With this new date on my calendar, my disappointment at being stood up was soon forgotten. I'm not saying that I can always get a date within an hour, but when I need to I can usually get a date within a few weeks with someone I am excited about. It wasn't always this way.

Many years ago, I met women through my friends. When my friends didn't fix me up, I was out of luck. I didn't know how to meet a woman on my own. It was such a helpless feeling, waiting month after month, not knowing when, if ever, I would have a girlfriend again. When a friend introduced me to the woman I eventually married, I hadn't had a date in over a year.

I met my coauthor Roger shortly after my sixteen-year marriage ended. At that time I was no better at meeting women than before I married. I was afraid I was in for another long period of loneliness. I wondered how Roger was doing—it had been three years since his divorce. When I asked him if he was dating anyone, he said, "I'm dating three women and I have the numbers of fourteen others in my little black book." I was impressed. I thought, "This guy isn't any better looking than me, we're both just average-looking guys, yet he has all those numbers and I don't have one. If he can do it, maybe I can too."

Encouraged by Roger's success, I decided to try to make something happen rather than just wait for a friend to fix me up. I decided to learn how to meet women. It wasn't easy. Going out to places where I might meet a woman didn't bother me, but actually walking up to a woman, starting a conversation, and asking her out scared me to death. This strong fear of rejection led me to look in places where I thought I would get rejected the least, such as singles bars, singles dances, and other singles functions. I felt that most of the women at singles places were there trying to meet men, so if I did get up the nerve to ask for a date, the odds are I would probably be asking a woman who was available.

When I think about the first year or so after my divorce, I'm amused at how inept I was at the meeting process. For example, in order to avoid the possibility of being rejected, instead of asking a woman out, I would give her my card and ask her to call. There was no immediate rejection with this method because all the women accepted my card with a smile. Not one woman called, however. Naturally I thought they didn't like me. One night I managed to work up the nerve to directly ask a woman for a date. When she accepted, I was amazed. I had learned the hard way that giving a woman my number and asking her to call doesn't work.

Over the years, as Roger and I were in and out of relationships, we continually tried new techniques and analyzed our experiences. Eventually, with the help of Diana (our friend and coauthor), we developed a step-by-step system for meeting the opposite sex that can be used successfully by both men and women. If *I* can learn this system and get over my fear of asking for a date, there is hope for almost anyone. Luckily, you don't have to spend years learning to meet the opposite sex as we did. You can benefit from our many years of experience and our in-depth analysis of the meeting process and become successful at meeting women in a much shorter time.

I am currently in a long-term relationship with a woman I met in a Western dance bar using the techniques described in this book. She is smart (a Ph.D.), pretty, and lots of fun. I'm getting spoiled by the way she treats me. Before I met her, I was casually dating three women and had dozens of other numbers. Years earlier, when I was thinking, "If Roger can do it, maybe I can too," I could only dream that I would someday master the meeting process. I have mastered the process, and with our help, you can too. The time to start is now.

ROGER'S STORY

I could tell Dave was impressed by my dating three women and having fourteen numbers in my little black book. At that time, I was impressed too. In retrospect, however, not one of those women was a good match for me, and I was in and out of relationships for several more years.

Over time I began to develop a better understanding of what I really wanted in a woman and realized that I might have to meet a fair number of women in order to find a good match. I also realized that meeting a woman who met my requirements was not just a matter of luck—it was something I could have considerable control over.

I wanted to meet an athletic and outdoor-loving woman, so I eventually concentrated on frequenting outdoor places and activities, especially bike paths and running events. Knowing that such a woman could be almost anywhere, however, I also took advantage of opportunities to meet women while running errands and traveling on business. I developed expertise at meeting women in such places as airplanes, the post office, and grocery stores. I found that the steps required to meet a woman in a nonsingles place such as a bike path or onboard an airplane are the same steps required at a typical singles place. The basic steps of the meeting process are pretty much the same everywhere.

I often try to help my single friends by recommending the same techniques I use; however, I usually get a reaction such as, "I'm not that desperate!" This reaction is hard for me to understand. If you want someone in your life, it just makes sense to try to make it happen. Being desperate has nothing to do with it.

I am now married to a woman I met on a bike path using the techniques recommended in this book. She is athletic, a vegetarian (like me), and an outdoor and fitness buff. We got married on a snowy winter day at the summit of Mount Elbert, which at 14,433 feet is the highest mountain in Colorado. The hike to the top and back was sixteen miles on snowshoes, with a five-thousand-foot vertical gain. Finding a woman who likes this kind of strenuous outdoor activity was not luck; I made it happen using the system described in this book—a system anyone can learn.

DIANA'S STORY

When I signed up for Dave and Roger's class "Meeting Men Made Easy," I had been divorced just a few months, and I was at a loss as to how to meet a man. The straightforward and useful advice they gave in that class turned out to be exactly what I needed. They made me realize that there was hope after all. Although at that time I felt that I didn't have the nerve to do everything they recommended, at least I finally knew what needed to be done—I had some direction.

I stayed after the class to talk with Dave and Roger. They seemed genuinely interested in the problems I was having meeting men, and they welcomed my comments on their class. Because it was late, they suggested that I meet them for dinner the next day to continue our discussion. I think Dave and Roger had an ulterior motive when they extended their dinner invitation. They wanted to get a woman's in-depth opinion on what they were teaching. I had an ulterior motive too: I wanted more help with my goal of finding a good man.

Our dinner conversation turned out to be beneficial for all, and dinner together became a regular event. Later, after I had become adept at using the techniques for meeting men that they had taught me, I started helping them teach their classes. Eventually I helped them write this book and our companion book, *How to Meet the Right Man*.

I can tell you from a woman's perspective, that the advice in this book makes sense. Women want to be approached by a man who is confident and interested in meeting them—it is a compliment. A confident man who knows what he is doing is appealing.

How We Began Teaching Others

We (Dave and Roger) have been meeting for lunch several times a week for the past ten years. Our favorite topic to discuss during these lunchtime bull sessions is how men and women meet. As you would expect from two engineers, we have analyzed the meeting process to death. We have spent hundreds of hours discussing the best places for singles to meet, what approaches work best, and the fears holding people back. After several years of our talks and discussions with other singles, we began to wonder if anyone in the world had analyzed the meeting process more than we had. We joked about writing a book or teaching a class on the subject. Several years ago, on a lark, we started teaching a class for men called "Meeting Women Made Easy." Preparing for that class forced us to organize our techniques into an easy-to-learn five-step format.

After several months of teaching this class for men, we started teaching a class for women called "Meeting Men Made Easy." Diana was a student in one of our early classes for women. Eventually she became a friend and joined us in teaching our classes. Diana provided the needed woman's perspective for our teaching and writing.

Eventually we combined the class for men and the class for women into one class for both men and women. Over the years we have taught hundreds of men and women ranging in age from teenagers to retirees. Some wanted to learn how to meet the opposite sex so they could get married and raise a family, while others just wanted companionship. High school and college students, blue-collar workers, white-collar workers, and professionals have all found our classes helpful.

In this book we teach how to meet a woman in a face-to-face situation. This method is our area of expertise. There are dozens of good books on getting psychologically prepared for going out to meet someone and, once you meet someone, how to have a good relationship. There is a big gap left by these books, however; they seldom cover the practical skills and knowledge needed to meet a woman and arrange a date—something that obviously must be accomplished before any relationship can begin. This book fills that gap.

All the stories in this book are true. Names have been changed for the usual reasons.

Part I

Empowering Yourself With the Facts

1

The Five Steps

When teaching our class "Meeting Women Made Easy," we start by saying, "Our method for getting a date is to walk up to a woman, start a conversation, and then ask her out. How many of you find this a new and exciting way to meet women?" Nobody ever raises a hand. They all know that is a way to meet women. Then we say, "Oh, that's too bad. You spent your money and drove all the way down here tonight, and you already know the method we teach."

At that point we hold up a poster of a gorgeous young blonde in a bikini. It's a white bikini decorated with sensuous red kisses. The poster is signed, *Love and Kisses—Janis*. As we walk around the room giving each man a close-up view of Janis, we say, "Imagine this scenario: You are in the supermarket when Janis runs into the store in her bikini to get some suntan lotion. How many of you would walk up to Janis, start a conversation, and then ask her out?" Nobody would ever raise a hand. Then we say, "We're confused. We thought you knew this method for meeting women. Is there something wrong with Janis? Isn't she cute? Why wouldn't you try to get a date with her?" This last question always gets a response out of the men, and their responses are always variations of, "I can't because I'm afraid."

You are a rare man indeed if you haven't felt this fear. It is a feeling so strong that it immobilizes many men when they see a desirable woman and think about meeting her. This fear, often called the "fear of rejection," is real, and it can make approaching a woman and asking for a date extremely difficult.

This book teaches a simple way to reduce this fear. It is a method that allows you to salami-slice the meeting process into smaller, less intimidating steps. To get an idea of how this is done, let's look at a true story about how Robert, a student of ours, got a date at the zoo. We will derive the basic steps for meeting a woman from what he did.

This story is not about Robert's first attempt to meet a woman at the zoo. He had previously tried to meet women at the zoo after reading a book that said the zoo was a good place to meet women. He told us about his first experience trying to meet a woman at the zoo:

> When I got to the zoo, I felt that the book had let me down. It hadn't said a thing about what to do once inside the zoo. Once I passed through the turnstile, I was on my own. I wandered around a while and then left. It was a waste of time.

After his failed attempt to meet a woman at the zoo, Robert took our class. We gave him a framework that he could use to meet a woman anywhere. Here is how he used that framework during his second attempt to meet a woman at the zoo.

> The first thing I did when I got to the zoo was look at the map by the entrance to see how the zoo was laid out. I wanted to make sure I followed a route that would let me cover the entire zoo. The location of the various animal exhibits wasn't important in my route selection. I was only interested in seeing the women who were at the zoo at that particular time.
>
> I walked my selected route at a brisk pace, making sure I passed through every bird, reptile, and animal house. I made a thorough search, being careful to include the concession stands and picnic areas. I was looking for an appealing woman who was either alone or with children and who appeared to be single. After making a complete tour of the zoo without seeing

such a woman, I returned to the entrance and sat on a bench where I could watch women as they came in.

After a short wait, an appealing woman and a young girl (who I assumed was her daughter) pushed through the turnstiles. The woman was wearing shorts and a halter top. When they passed by, I could see that she wasn't wearing a wedding ring, and I noticed she had a gold chain bracelet around her ankle. I decided to try to meet her.

The two of them set off toward the first animal exhibit, and I casually headed in the same direction. When they stopped at the first exhibit, they were in the middle of a crowd. Since there was no room for me to get near her, I waited. At the next exhibit she stood at a railing watching the chimpanzees. This time there was plenty of room, so I moved up to the railing and looked at the chimpanzees.

I had an icebreaker ready. I was going to say, "Did you know this animal is extinct?" I knew it sounded stupid, but I also knew it would get a reaction that might start a conversation. However, I was curious about her ankle bracelet. I had heard that some girls wear an ankle bracelet to show they're going steady. I decided to change my icebreaker so I could find out if that was what her ankle chain meant. I turned to her and said, "Do you know why a primate would wear a gold chain around its ankle?" She glanced at me and then back at the chimpanzees and replied, "Sometimes they band these animals." With a big grin, I pointed at the bracelet around her ankle and said, "What does *that* mean?" Laughing at my joke, she said, "Oh that! It doesn't mean anything. I just like to wear my ankle chain when I wear shorts."

When I introduced myself, she said that her name was Janet and her daughter's name was Crystal. I asked Crystal where she went to school and what grade she was in. I mentioned I had a son in the same grade. We made light conversation for a minute or so, but it was sort of awkward talking there in front of the chimpanzee cage where the crowd was now pressing around us. Janet looked uneasy, as if she didn't know if she should break off the conversation and move on. To get us all out of this uncomfortable situation, I offered to buy a round of ice cream cones. Crystal's face lit up and she looked up at her mother expectantly. Janet accepted my offer with a smile.

While we were seated at a picnic table eating our ice cream, I learned that Janet was divorced. She also told me that she was a dental hygienist, working with Dr. John Anderson, a dentist on Pearl Street.

We talked until we had finished our ice cream. By then, I knew I wanted to see her again, so I asked her if we could meet for lunch during the coming week. She said Tuesday would be best for her. She gave me her work number and suggested that I call her on Monday to arrange the details of the date. It was apparent that her daughter wanted to get on with their tour of the zoo, so I excused myself by saying I had some yard work waiting for me at home.

Robert used the Five-Step process for meeting a woman that we had taught in our class. Here are the Five Steps Robert took that resulted in his getting a date with Janet:

Step 1—Search

If Robert had spent his afternoon at the zoo strolling from exhibit to exhibit looking at the animals, it would have been pure luck if an appealing and available woman had appeared beside him. Instead, Robert took control of the situation by making a special effort to search for a woman to meet. His search consisted of a moving phase where he quickly toured the entire zoo to see who was there, and then a stationary phase where he sat and watched who came in. Robert spent his time looking for a woman, not looking at the animals.

Step 2—Get Near

After Robert found a woman he wanted to meet, he moved with the crowd, waiting for an opportunity to get next to her. When he saw an opening at the railing in front of the chimpanzee cage, he walked over, stood beside her, and looked at the chimpanzees. He was then near enough to say something.

Step 3—Break the Ice

Robert had an icebreaker ready to use. No matter what animal exhibit a woman was in front of, he planned to say, "Did you know this animal is extinct?" It was a silly opener, but he felt it would get a reaction. When he saw Janet's gold ankle bracelet, however, he decided not to use his planned icebreaker. His joke about a primate with an ankle chain served to get the conversation started and at the same time let him know if the ankle bracelet had any romantic significance.

Step 4—Continue the Conversation

After introducing himself, Robert sustained the conversation during its first critical moments by asking questions about Janet's daughter. By asking where Crystal went to school, Robert was able to quickly eliminate the possibility that Janet and Crystal were from out of town. Knowing where Crystal went to school told him approximately where in the metropolitan area they lived. When talking in front of the chimpanzee cage became awkward after a few minutes, he offered to buy ice cream.

While the three enjoyed their ice cream, Robert kept the conversation going by talking about Janet's job. He made a point of finding out the name of the dentist she worked with. This information would allow him to call her at work in case he failed, for any number of reasons, to ask her out during their first meeting at the zoo.

Step 5—Close

Robert closed by asking Janet if she could meet him for lunch.

Robert's ability to get a date with Janet was not the result of any one action or a cute "line." He was successful because he took five sequential actions (the Five Steps) that each increased his chance to meet, and get a date with, a woman he found attractive.

WHY THESE FIVE STEPS?

These are the basic steps every man goes through when meeting a woman in a face-to-face situation. We didn't invent these steps. They became apparent to us when we analyzed the meeting process. Thinking in terms of these Five Steps has several advantages:

- ◆ You have a framework for planning what to do in different situations.
- ◆ You can reduce your fear by focusing on one small step at a time instead of the entire process of approaching a woman and asking for a date.
- ◆ If you can isolate your biggest problem getting dates as a single step, you can concentrate on getting better at that step.

Let's look at the Five Steps again. We will examine the purpose of each step and give more details on how each step can be applied. Once you understand the purpose of each step, you will have a basis for determining how to apply that particular step in different situations.

The explanation of these steps assumes that you are at a place where there are women (singles dance, store, lecture, baseball game, etc.). Whether you are at a typical singles meeting place such as a singles mixer or singles bar or at a nonsingles place such as a store or bike path does not matter. The steps apply equally well to both singles and nonsingles meeting situations.

STEP 1—SEARCH

Purpose
Select the woman (or women) you want to meet.

The process of meeting a woman starts when you select, from all those available, one or more women that you find attractive and want to meet. If you don't search, you generally limit your selection to just the few women who happen to be close by. Searching allows you to select from all the women who are there.

Different places require different search strategies. The search strategy in a singles bar will be different from the search strategy in a shopping mall. A good search strategy at a ski slope may not make sense at a 10K run. There are some common principles, however, that govern when and how to search.

When to Search

If you are going to a place where you will be spending most of your time fixed in one spot, such as a lecture, a night school class, or an opera, the most effective search strategy is to go early and watch women as they arrive. When an appealing and apparently unattached woman arrives and takes a seat, take a seat near her or next to her. That puts you in a position where it will be easy to start a conversation. If your search before the event isn't successful, you can search again during the breaks and immediately after the event.

If you are going to an event where you can move about, such as a library or city park, when you arrive is not critical because you can search effectively whenever you arrive. Arriving when it is crowded gives you more women to choose from.

How to Search

The best search strategy depends on whether the women are fixed in one spot or moving about. If the women are stationary, you must move about to see who is there. For example, at a summer concert in the park, most people take a blanket or chair and sit in one spot for the entire concert. In a situation such as that, you will have your best chance of seeing a variety of women by moving from one location to another. At an event where people are moving about, you can either remain in one spot and watch women walk by, move around yourself, or alternate between these two methods. For example, at an amusement park, people will be continually moving from one ride or concession stand to another. You could search by sitting on a bench and watching women pass by, by walking through the amusement park, or by alternating between these two strategies.

STEP 2—GET NEAR

Purpose

To get within speaking distance of the woman you want to meet.

You can't get a date with a woman without talking to her first, and to talk to her you must be near enough to speak. In most situations, the man most likely to meet a woman is the man closest to her. Put yourself in that position.

In some situations, such as when a woman is standing alone away from a crowd, it would be awkward for both of you if you were to walk over and stand close to her without saying something. In such situations you must be prepared to say something as soon as you get near. There are many other situations, however, where you have the option of getting near a woman without immediately speaking to her. This is especially easy to do in places that are fairly crowded, such as at sit-down events, or at stores and malls where you can get near a woman as you both go about your business.

If you are afraid to approach an attractive woman and try to get a date (as most men are), it really helps to concentrate on the step of first getting near, without giving any thought to what you are going to do next. Don't pile one stressful step immediately on top of another—it might become more of a challenge than you can handle. Even though you may not know what you are going to say to a woman, you can still get near her. Don't stand there looking across the room at a woman, agonizing over how you will ever meet her. Instead, say to yourself, "I must find a way to get near her." Sometimes, without any additional effort, you will meet her just because you are near. Perhaps she will turn to *you* and ask a question, or there may be something that happens nearby that you can comment on as an icebreaker. No matter who speaks first, you must be near for anything to happen.

Getting near is a step that's easy to practice. Whenever you see an appealing woman, try to go near her. Don't worry about the rest of the Five Steps. Taking action only on this step will result in your meeting more women.

STEP 3—BREAK THE ICE

Purpose

To get a conversation started.

Some men feel that if they only had the "right" line, the perfect icebreaker, meeting a woman would suddenly become easy. For example, we are frequently asked by men in our class, "What do you say to meet a woman in the supermarket?" The men who ask that question seem to feel that the only thing standing in their way of meeting those desirable women in the supermarket is the lack of a perfect icebreaker. When we suggest several icebreakers they could use at the supermarket, however, they always seem disappointed. The reason is simple: There is no magic icebreaker that will eliminate their fear—and it is fear, not the lack of a perfect icebreaker, that keeps men from starting conversations with women.

Witty remarks, "lines," and "perfect" icebreakers are not necessary for starting a conversation with a woman in a supermarket, or anywhere else for that matter. If the woman is somewhat open to meeting you, almost anything you say will get a conversation going. On the other hand, if she wants to be left alone, nothing you say is likely to work. But you do need to say *something* to find out which of these two women she is. The one critical rule for starting a conversation with a woman is: *Anything you say is better than saying nothing.*

Since you do need to say *something*, it can help enormously to know what that something is going to be. You need to plan icebreakers that you can use in a given situation. The simple fact that you have something ready to say will make you more confident.

Planned Icebreakers

If you wait until you see an appealing woman before thinking of an icebreaker, your stress level may be so high that you won't be able to come up with one. Plan ahead so you will be certain to have something to say. You might come up with one icebreaker that will work no matter where you meet a woman or what she is doing, or several that will cover a range of situations that you are likely to encounter.

Going to the same type of event again and again and not know-ing what to say to start a conversation is a sure sign that you need to plan a couple of icebreakers. And don't wait until you have the perfect icebreaker that you think will make meeting women easy—it's not the icebreaker that makes meeting women easy, it's practice. Come up with some icebreakers and go with them.

Here are some examples of planned icebreakers. These may or may not appeal to you. You need to come up with icebreakers that you will be comfortable with.

At a shopping mall: "Only 250 shopping days till Christmas. Are you ready?"

At an art gallery: "Do you like this artist's work?"

Walking beside a woman on a downtown street: "This is a nice day to be out. Are you on your lunch hour?"

At an intermission during a lecture: "What do you think of the talk so far?"

At some places there could be a small number of different activities that a woman might be engaged in. In this situation, you can plan appropriate icebreakers for each of the activities. For example, at a supermarket you might see a woman engaged in one of the follow-ing activities:

♦ Pushing her cart down the aisle
♦ Looking at some canned or packaged goods
♦ Picking out a fruit or vegetable
♦ Standing in line at the checkout counter

You could plan icebreakers in advance to cover all of these likely situations:

She is pushing her cart down the aisle. You pull up alongside of her and say:
"Did you get a wobbly wheel cart today?"

She is looking at canned goods. You take a can off the shelf and say:
"Do you know what these numbers on the bar code mean?"

She is selecting some fruit or vegetable. You say:
"How do you pick a good [canteloupe, avocado, squash, pineapple, etc.]?"

She is in the checkout line. You say:
"What do you think—did we pick the slowest line?"

With these four planned icebreakers you have some likely situations in a grocery store covered. If our examples do not appeal to you, make up your own.

Spontaneous Icebreakers

Even though you have a planned icebreaker ready, when you see a woman you want to meet, be open to spur-of-the-moment, "spontaneous" icebreakers. Spontaneous icebreakers relate to something about the woman or your immediate situation or surroundings. If you come up with a spontaneous icebreaker and like it, you have the option of using it instead of your planned icebreaker. If you don't come up with something you like, you have your planned icebreaker to fall back on.

Here are examples of spontaneous icebreakers:

At a shopping mall—to a woman carrying a lot of packages:
"You are certainly helping the economy."

At an art gallery—to a woman wearing a silk scarf with a beautiful print:
"Your scarf should be on display here. The colors are beautiful."

At a supermarket—to a woman with cat food in her cart:
"What kind of cat do you have?"

A man who has conquered his fear doesn't agonize over what he is going to say to a woman to start a conversation. He walks up to a woman and starts talking, just as he would if she were his sister or next-door neighbor. Until you have conquered your fear, however, it does help to have a planned icebreaker. This is a confidence booster that will increase the chance that you will say something when the opportunity arises.

STEP 4—CONTINUE THE CONVERSATION

Purpose

To have a relaxed conversation directed toward achieving specific goals.

After you have started a conversation, you need to continue it for a comfortable period of time. During this time you are gathering important information and deciding if you want to ask the woman out. Although conversation might be easy for you under most circumstances, the emotional turmoil you feel in the presence of an appealing woman can make you freeze up. One way to avoid getting tongue-tied is to guide the conversation so that you can achieve specific conversation goals. We recommend the following three conversation goals. These goals will help you keep a conversation going while at the same time giving you valuable information about the woman.

Conversation Goal No. 1—Get Insurance

"Insurance" is our shorthand term for a useful concept. Insurance consists of the woman's name and at least enough information about where she works to enable you to look up her company's phone number and call her there. This information is your "insurance" that in case your conversation gets interrupted, you will still be able to get in touch with her in the future.

Obviously, having a woman's first and last name gives you the best insurance because you can look her up in the phone book and, if she is listed, call her at home. Her full name also makes it easier to reach her at work. To get her full name, introduce yourself with both your first and last names. She will usually respond by giving you her first and last names.

The only downside to getting a woman's full name is that it might be difficult to remember both her first and last names, and it's usually the last name that is forgotten only moments after a conversation begins. To remember her full name, use her first name when talking to her, and make her last name the first topic of conversation. You can discuss such things as the spelling of her last name, its origin, or how attractive a name it is. For example, you could say:

"Schawinski. Is that s-k-i or s-k-y?"

"Doucette—that's French, isn't it?"

"Mary Martinez! What a pretty name."

In addition to her name, find out where she works so you can call her there if the need arises. The amount of information you will need to reach her at work depends on the size of her company. For example, if she tells you that her name is Betty and she's the secretary for Distinctive Real Estate Company, you probably have enough information to be able to reach her at work. If her name is Betty and she's a secretary for the Internal Revenue Service, however, you aren't going to have much luck calling the IRS and asking for Betty.

When a woman works for a large organization such as the IRS, to be able to reach her at work when you only have her first name, you need more information about the kind of work she does and the department she is in. By asking her questions about her work, eventually you should have enough information to be able to reach her with the help of the company operator and the person who answers the phone in her department. For instance, if you learn that Betty is a technical editor at the IRS office in your city, and you know that she works in the Publications Department, you could probably call the IRS, ask for the Publications Department, and then ask for Betty who works as a technical editor.

Insurance is useful for those situations where your conversation gets interrupted and you can't close. Although insurance is useful as a backup, it's too risky to use as your primary method of getting a woman's number. Here's Frank's story about how he depended too heavily on insurance:

When I left the dance, I was feeling pretty good about myself because I had done a smooth job of meeting Mary. I had seen her turning men down when they asked her to dance, and although I felt I would probably get the same treatment, I asked her anyway. To my surprise, she accepted my offer. As we were dancing, I started right in on a conversation. She told me that her name was Mary and she worked in the land department at American Petroleum. When I asked her what she did in the land department, she told me that she was a contract analyst. At that point I felt I could reach her by calling American Petroleum, asking for the land department, and then asking to speak to Mary the contract analyst. I wanted to ask Mary for a date while I was dancing with her, but just couldn't get up the nerve. Since I felt I could call her at work on Monday and ask her out, I didn't struggle too hard to get my nerve up.

On Monday, when I called American Petroleum, things came unraveled pretty fast. The company telephone operator put me through to the land department okay, but when a woman answered the phone and I asked for Mary the contract analyst, this woman said, "Sir, we have over three hundred people in this department and we have forty-six contract analysts. I don't know them all. If you can't give me a last name, I can't help you." I said, "Oh," and hung up. I wish I had asked Mary out while I was dancing with her.

Frank used insurance as his primary method of asking for a date, but this time it didn't work. After this incident, he started asking women out while he was face-to-face with them.

Conversation Goal No. 2—Qualify Her

When you see a woman for the first time, her appearance is all you can judge her on. The initial conversation is an opportunity to find out more about the complete package, so you can judge whether or not she is right for you.

What are you looking for in a woman? Is her religion important to you? Are you looking for someone who will share your interest in a hobby or activity? Would you object if she had children? How far would you be willing to travel to see her? Once you define what you want and need in a woman, these requirements can help you "qualify" a potential partner during your initial conversation to see if she matches your needs. When you qualify a woman, you get information to help you decide how long to talk to her and whether to ask for a date.

The questions you ask in order to qualify a woman will help keep the conversation rolling; however, *how* you ask these questions is important. If you ask the questions in quick succession, the woman will probably feel as if she is being interviewed—something she might find objectionable. A good way to obtain the information you need is to ask a question and then follow it up with some additional conversation on that topic. You want to weave your questions into the conversation so she won't feel as if she is being interrogated.

Direct questions are not always necessary. For example, saying, "They should raise the tax on cigarettes by a dollar a pack," is almost sure to get a reaction that will tell you whether she smokes or not. Simply bringing up a topic and watching her reaction can tell you a lot.

Jim is one of the men who took our class. He is divorced and has two children in college and a lot of free time. Let's see what Jim's requirements are and how he uses them to qualify the women he meets. Here is what Jim told us about the type of woman he was looking for:

> My favorite activities are jogging, backpacking, and bike riding. My ideal outing is to drive up to the mountains on Friday after work, sleep in the car, and then backpack in for the weekend. I'm looking for a woman who enjoys this type of strenuous outdoor life and who has most weekends free to travel with me.

We provide our students with a form for listing their requirements. Jim's filled-out form shows his requirements for the woman he wants to meet (see page 18).

The Type of Woman I Want to Meet

Category	Jim's Requirements
Age	No preset age restrictions.
Marital History	I don't care if she is divorced or never married.
Children	Okay if she has kids, but not full responsibility for them. I want her to be able to go away some weekends.
Religion	I would prefer her not to be religious.
Geographic	No great restrictions, just so we can get together on the weekends.
Smoking	Nonsmoker a must.
Drinking	No heavy drinkers.
Drug Use	No drug users.
Education	Not of great importance but prefer college education.
Occupation	Not critical but prefer her to have a professional job.
Financial Status	The more money the better, but it's not really important.
Character	She must not be a homebody (a quiet evening at home drives me nuts).
Type of Relationship	I want a long-term relationship but have no great desire to get married.
Interests	Must share my interest in outdoor activities such as hiking. Must like to travel.

A month after he took our class, Jim came to one of the support group meetings we hold for our students. At that meeting, Jim described how he was using his requirements as a guide to help him determine if a woman was right for him:

> I qualify a woman even before I talk to her. I get a lot of information just by looking at her clothes and makeup. If she is heavily made up and perfumed, has long painted fingernails, and is a flashy dresser, I don't have much hope she's going to enjoy my lifestyle. For me, good signs are a casual, natural look. Running shoes, shorts or jeans, and a backpack are all good signs.
>
> Once I begin a conversation with a woman, I start qualifying her within the first few minutes. One of the first things I do is try to find out if her job would keep her from getting away on weekends. Here are some of the questions I usually ask, and actual answers I have gotten:

> ME: "What kind of work do you do?"
> WOMAN NO. 1: "I don't have a full-time job. I'm a student at the art institute and work weekends at a print shop." (*Not good. She's probably busy studying during the week and working on weekends.*)
> WOMAN NO. 2: "I'm a secretary for Tri-County Electric." (*Good sign. She probably works a normal Monday-through-Friday schedule and could get away on weekends.*)

> If the woman says she has children, I try to find out if she has full responsibility for them:

> ME: "You said you have a three-year-old son. Does his father see him very often?"
> WOMAN NO. 1: "No, he's been living out of state since our divorce and hasn't seen Brian in over a year." (*Bad sign. She probably has full responsibility for her son every weekend.*)

WOMAN NO. 2: "Yes, he lives nearby and takes them every other weekend." (*Good! Sounds as if she might be able to get away pretty often.*)

I also ask questions to find out how active she is:

ME: "What did you do today?"
WOMAN NO. 1: "Not much—just watched TV." (*What a slug. Imagine watching TV on such a beautiful day.*)
WOMAN NO. 2: "I went for a bike ride with my girlfriend." (*Good sign. She could be interesting.*)

Jim followed his program and eventually met a woman on the bike path who turned out to be a great companion. The last time we talked to Jim, he and Sharon had just gotten back from a vacation in Guatemala. They had spent a week exploring Mayan ruins and hiking through remote Indian villages.

Qualifying a woman early in a conversation can save you time. You are going to talk about something when you first meet—it might as well be about things that are important to you. You don't have to spend an entire evening with a woman learning whether or not she meets your basic requirements. You can find out in the first twenty minutes or so.

The advantage to qualifying a woman in the first few minutes of conversation is that if she doesn't meet some of your important requirements, you can spend your time finding a woman who does. Al, a student of ours, learned that lesson the hard way.

I had an experience at a benefit dance that taught me a valuable lesson about asking the right questions. I had asked this woman, Julie, to dance. As we danced, we talked about her family, what she did for a living, and what she liked to do for fun. We seemed to hit it off right away. I liked her a lot, and we danced and talked for the entire evening. At midnight I asked Julie for a date and she agreed to go out. When I asked for her address so I could pick her up, she told me she lived in Larkspur—a three-hour drive from where I lived. I was extremely disappointed. I thought that was too far to drive. At that point, I backed out of the date with a sincere apology. Julie said she understood because she had run into the same problem with other men.

Al wasted the entire evening because early in their conversation he failed to ask Julie the simple question, "Where do you live?"

Before you can come up with the questions you should ask to find out if a woman meets your requirements, you need to have a pretty good idea what your requirements are. To help you think about what your most important requirements are, we have provided a blank requirements form in Appendix A like the one Jim filled out. This form might help you establish what you are really looking for in a woman.

Conversation Goal No. 3—Extend Your Time Together

In some situations, it is acceptable to ask for a date after only a brief conversation. For example, it is usually not necessary to have a two hour conversation with a woman at a singles bar or a singles social event before asking her out. Most women go to singles activities hoping to meet a man, and your request for a date after only ten or fifteen minutes of conversation should not come as a shock. In places that are not typical singles places, however, asking for a date after only a few minutes of conversation might seem too abrupt. If you were to meet a woman at a business seminar and ask her out too soon, she might turn you down because your request was unexpected or because it seemed inappropriate. One way to ease into the possibility of romance is to "extend your time together" by asking her to go somewhere with you right now. At a seminar, for example, you might suggest that the two of you go somewhere for coffee or for a short walk outside to get some fresh air. After this additional time together, asking for a date will be more appropriate.

Extending your time together is also useful when you are in a situation where you might get interrupted at any minute or where it's awkward to talk for an extended time. Say you are in a bookstore and you have been talking with a woman for about ten minutes, and the two of you seem to be hitting it off, but it is getting awkward standing there. You also feel that it would be difficult to ask her out with other people standing so close by. In this situation, a suggestion to get a cup of coffee next door is perfect. If she accepts, you have an indication that she is interested in you. Once you are in a booth at the coffee shop having coffee together, you will have more time to get to know one another, and the setting will be much more comfortable for a long conversation. If you then decide that you still want to see her again, the setting will be more private, and that should make it easier to ask her out.

STEP 5—CLOSE

Purpose

To get her phone number.

In sales jargon, "close" means to finalize the sale. In regard to getting a date, "close" means to get a woman's phone number. You can just get her phone number, or you can arrange a date and get her phone number. In either case, it is the phone number that allows you to reach her again.

This step is the one that gives you the ability to start a relationship. Below are some effective ways to get a phone number. Pick the one that suits you the best. There doesn't seem to be a consensus among women as to which is most preferable.

Directly Ask If you Can Call Her

Many women have had the experience of giving their number to a man and not being called. Therefore, avoid saying, "Could I have your number?" Instead, ask for her number in a way that emphasizes that you intend to call. For example, you could say:

"Would it be okay if I called you?"

"Could I call you when I get back from my trip on Thursday?"

"Could I call you tomorrow at work?"

Once you get a woman's number, call when you said you would and arrange a date. If you didn't tell her when you would call, then call within a day or two. She will appreciate an early call so she can stop wondering whether or not she will ever hear from you.

Some women will refuse to give you their number and will ask for yours instead. What happens then? Does she call? Usually not. It's not necessarily because she doesn't like you or doesn't want to see you again. She may simply be uncomfortable at the thought of calling a man.

Diane told us how she felt about calling a man she met at a run.

After Tim and I had talked for a while at the run, he asked for my number. I wanted to stay in control, so I didn't give it to him. I got his instead, and I promised him I would call. It wasn't easy making that call. I don't like to call men I don't know very well, so I kept putting it off. Besides, I had the feeling that he might not really have wanted to go out with me and was just going through the motions by asking for my number. After a couple of days, so much time had gone by that I was afraid if I called, he would answer the phone and say, "Who?" If my daughter hadn't insisted that I start getting out of the house more, I would never have called him.

When a woman refuses to give you her number and asks for yours instead, emphasize that you really want her to call you. You can also increase the chances that she will call by suggesting a time when she could call. For example, you could say, "I'll be cleaning my house tomorrow morning; that would be a good time for you to call." Suggest a time that is within a day or so. The further away the suggested time is, the less likely it is that she will call.

Ask for a Date "Sometime"

You can ask a woman if she would like to go out sometime, and not specify a certain time or activity. The advantage of asking for a date "sometime" rather than for a specific time and place is that she won't say, "Oh, I'm busy that night," which would leave you wondering whether she does or does not want to go out with you. Here are some ways to ask a woman to go out "sometime."

"Would you like to go out sometime?"

"Would you like to play racquetball sometime?"

"Would you like to get together for lunch sometime?"

"Could we get together for a drink sometime?"

Once she agrees, get her number. You could say something like, "If you give me your number, I'll call you on Monday."

Ask for a Date, and Specify the Time and Place

You have the option of asking a woman to join you for a specific activity at a specific time. When suggesting such a date, be prepared to offer an alternative in case she can't make it for some reason. If she refuses your initial offer, follow up with something like, "Would you like to get together at another time?" Here are some examples of asking for a date that is for a specific activity at a specific time:

"Could we meet for lunch next Tuesday at Maxwell's?"

"If I can get theater tickets for Saturday night, would you like to go?"

"It's supposed to be a nice day tomorrow; would you like to go for a bike ride?"

Ask for an Immediate Date

You don't have to suggest a date that is on another day. You can ask for a date for later that same day or for a date that you could go on immediately.

Asking for a date for the same day might seem like a bold approach, but it makes a lot of sense to use it. When two people meet and hit it off right away, there's no reason to wait several days before beginning the relationship. Asking for an immediate date or for a date later that day can make you seem exciting and spontaneous, someone who would be fun to know. Here are some typical scenarios where you could use this technique:

You have met a woman at a cocktail party: "This party is pretty dead. Would you be interested in going dancing?"

You are on a ski lift with a woman, and it is late in the day: "I know a great barbecue place in town. Would you like to get together later for dinner?"

You have met a woman at a Saturday-morning adult enrichment class: "Would you like to go for a bike ride this afternoon?"

Sometimes a woman will say she's busy when you ask for an date. When that happens, follow up with something like, "Would you like to make it another time?"

After You Have Arranged a Date, **Always Try to Get Her Phone Number**

It's possible to arrange a date without getting the woman's phone number, but when you do, you have not really closed. One reason you might be tempted to do this is because it reduces the chance of direct rejection. For example, you might be dancing with a woman in a singles bar and learn that she often comes there on Wednesday night. To avoid direct rejection, you close by saying, "Let's meet here next Wednesday and dance together again." If she shows up Wednesday, fine. If not, you are out of luck; you can't call her and arrange another date because you didn't get her number. You would have to go back every Wednesday, for who knows how long, before you would see her again and get another chance to ask her out.

Barry always gets a woman's number now, because he had a bad experience on one occasion when he didn't.

It was getting late, and I had been dancing with Sherry for half an hour. I thought it was time to ask her out. Since we were in a singles bar, I thought I should offer her a safe date where I would meet her somewhere. That way she wouldn't have to get in my car until she knew me better. So I asked her if she would like to meet me at the Silver Spur for some western dancing on Friday. She said that sounded like fun, so I told her I would meet her by the south entrance at eight-thirty. I didn't ask for her number because I was sure that I would make it, and if she wanted to stand me up, my having her number wouldn't change anything.

Friday morning it started snowing. By six o'clock that evening there was a foot of snow on the ground and a screaming blizzard. There was no way I could go the fifteen miles to the Silver Spur, and I couldn't imagine Sherry going either. It was a helpless feeling. I went there on the next night and stood by the south entrance, but she didn't show. I never saw her again.

If you arrange to meet a woman somewhere and don't get her number, in many cases something will go wrong and you won't see her again.

How Soon to Close

Do you need to spend two hours in conversation with a woman before you ask her out? In most situations, probably not. In a singles meeting situation, after ten or twenty minutes of conversation, you both probably know whether or not you are interested in a date. In a nonsingles meeting situation, however, given that you have the time, it is usually desirable to talk somewhat longer. For example, if you have started a conversation with a woman at an outdoor café, asking for a date in ten minutes may be too soon. Talking for a half hour or an hour might be more appropriate.

What if you have the choice of asking her out at another time? For example, say you are talking to a woman at a cocktail party and you think to yourself, "I will talk to her again later in the evening and ask her out then." That puts off having to face possible rejection, but it also reduces the chance that you will get a date. She might leave before you get to talk to her again, or she might talk to another man for the rest of the evening. As a general rule, "seize the moment" and close while you are with the woman during your first meeting.

If you want to get a date with a woman, in most situations you will have to complete the Five Steps. To ensure you will do these impor-

tant steps, before you go to a place or event, plan how you will execute each of the Five Steps in that environment. Having a plan will
give you more confidence, and confidence is the name of the game.

Another way to increase your confidence is to practice executing
at least some of the steps. Start with Step 1, searching, and do as
many as you can whenever you can as a friend of ours, George, did.
Here is what he told us.

When I got to the post office there was a crowd waiting, so I
took a number and waited to be called. As I looked around
the room, I saw a woman wearing a T-shirt that said CANCUN.
I felt real obvious as I worked my way over to her. When I got
next to her, I asked her if she had been to Cancun, and we got
to talking.

I intended to ask her out, but I felt I should talk to her as
long as I could before I did. I estimated that I had about five
minutes before her number would be called. About two minutes later, they called four numbers in quick succession and
nobody responded. Then they called her number and she was
gone.

All I knew about her was her first name, so I had no way to
reach her. I wished I had found out where she worked so I
could at least have had a shot at getting in touch with her again.
At least I felt good about myself for even starting a conversation with her. It wasn't as hard as I thought.

George wanted to get a date with the woman in the Cancun T-
shirt, but all he got was practice, some confidence building, and a
reminder to get insurance early in conversation.

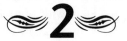

How to Avoid a No

The type of date you suggest can determine whether a woman you have just met will agree to go out with you. How do you know what type of date to suggest? We recommend that you consider the woman's point of view. Ask yourself three questions about the date you are about to suggest:

1. Will she feel safe?
2. Will she feel comfortable?
3. Will she be interested in the date activity?

WILL SHE FEEL SAFE?

Even if a woman likes you, she might not accept a date if it seems unsafe. For example, let's suppose you are at a singles dance, it's eleven at night, and you've been dancing and talking with a woman for about an hour. What do you suppose her reaction would be if you said, "How about hopping in my car and going over to Tommy's Diner for some dessert and coffee?" You might get a negative reaction, not because she doesn't like you, but because she doesn't want to get in a car late at night with a man she doesn't know very well.

At this point you may be thinking, "If a woman doesn't like the date I offered because it makes her feel unsafe, why doesn't she just make a counteroffer?" Some women might, but many won't. Most women aren't used to taking the initiative in arranging dates and won't be prepared to suggest a date that is more to their liking. Since you don't know what will cause anxiety in a particular woman, address as many safety issues in your offer as you can. Here are some recommendations:

Suggest a daytime activity: Daytime activities seem safer to most women.

Suggest a date at a well-known, busy public place: A bustling place she has heard of should cause few safety concerns.

Offer to pick her up, or to meet her there: Giving her this choice covers your bases. Some women are reluctant to get in a car with a man they don't know well, while others are offended if you don't offer to pick them up. Therefore, give her a choice by saying, "I can meet you there or pick you up, whichever you prefer."

Tip: *From a safety point of view, meeting for lunch at a popular restaurant is one of the best dates you can suggest. It is a daytime activity at a busy, well-known place, and she doesn't have to get in your car.*

Don't wait until you are in a meeting situation to determine what kind of date to suggest. Think it through ahead of time. If you come up with a date suggestion "on the fly" you may be missing something and setting yourself up for failure.

When Kevin met Maria, he offered a date that he thought she would consider safe. He hadn't thought it through from her perspective, however, Here is Kevin's story:

While I was dancing with Maria at a singles dance sponsored by a church, she mentioned how much she liked country dancing. I wanted to ask her out, and this gave me an idea for a date

I could suggest: I would ask her to go to Two Cowboys, a country dance spot. Since I was aware that some women are afraid to date the men they meet at singles events, I offered what I thought was a safe date. I didn't ask for her phone number, and I didn't offer to pick her up at her house. Instead, I arranged to meet her at Two Cowboys on Tuesday night.

I waited in Two Cowboys for an hour past our meeting time, but Maria didn't show up. Naturally, I thought I had been stood up. I assumed she didn't like me. However, some months later I ran into Maria and was surprised that she was so happy to see me. She explained what happened the night we were going to meet: "I drove over to Two Cowboys to meet you, but I hadn't realized that was such a tough part of town. The parking lot was full of beat-up pickup trucks. I didn't know if you were inside or not, and I was afraid to go in alone. I decided not to go in. I didn't have your number so I couldn't call you and explain what happened. I'm really sorry."

Maria didn't show up because Kevin had ignored some important safety issues. To meet him, Maria had to drive to a tough part of town at night, park in the parking lot, and walk into an unfamiliar bar alone. Kevin had set himself up for a no-show. And to make a bad situation worse, they had not traded phone numbers. Maria had no way to get in touch with him again. Lucky for him, they did meet again.

WILL SHE FEEL COMFORTABLE?

Some men think they need to impress a woman on the first date by offering dinner at an expensive restaurant, followed by some dancing, a movie, or a play. This full-blown formal Saturday night date may not be the best kind of date to offer, however. With some women, it can raise comfort issues. One issue is the length of the date. If a woman decides early in the evening that there is no chemistry, she will still have several more hours to carry on what could be a forced and awkward conversation. She also might be concerned about how and when to end the date, whether or not she should invite the man in, and what to do if he wants to get affectionate. A woman won't have these concerns with a short, informal date such as meeting for lunch or meeting for drinks after work. Does this mean you should always suggest a short, informal date? Not necessarily. Here is how two different women described a first date experience:

Woman No. 1

"We had arranged to go to an afternoon play, but then he turned it into a big fancy date. After the play we went to this expensive restaurant. He had made reservations and hadn't told me. I hate those long, formal dates when I'm not even sure I like the man. For a first date I prefer something simple."

Woman No. 2

"This guy was cheap! So cheap he only invited me out for lunch. I guess he didn't think I was worth a dinner."

So what's a man to do? Unless you have a good idea of what kind of date a particular woman would like, your best bet is to give her a choice. For example, you could say:

"Would you like to go out? Perhaps lunch or dinner sometime early next week?"

or

"How about getting together for a drink after work? Or maybe we could go to dinner instead. Either one is okay with me."

Offering both a simple, short date and a more elaborate date lets you get some feedback on her comfort zone. Once she expresses a preference, you can follow up on it and arrange the details, including getting her phone number.

Sometimes the safety issue and the comfort issue combine to

make a woman anxious about a prospective date. This happened to Kathy:

> Glenn and I met on a Sunday group hike and I liked him right away. At the end of the hike I was hoping he would ask me out, but I was caught off guard when he said, "Would you like to come over to my house next Saturday night? I'll cook dinner."
>
> I didn't like the idea of going to his house for dinner. He seemed nice, but I really didn't know him very well. I was in a quandary because I did want to see him again, and I didn't want to hurt his feelings by acting as if I didn't trust him. I agreed to the date, but with serious misgivings.
>
> All week I worried about the date I had agreed to. I called three of my girlfriends and asked them what I should do. Several times I thought about canceling. I did end up going, and there weren't any problems. He's a nice guy, but going to his house on the first date sure caused me a lot of concern.

When Glenn offered to cook dinner at his place, he was trying to impress Kathy. He considered himself a good cook and was proud of his well-decorated home in a prestigious neighborhood. By concentrating on impressing Kathy and not on thinking about her concerns, he almost got a rejection.

Will She Be Interested in the Date Activity?

If possible, offer an activity that you know she likes. You have an opportunity to find out what a woman likes when you qualify her during your initial conversation. For example, you could ask, "What do you like to do in your spare time?" or "What do you do for fun?" Then when you ask for a date, capitalize on what you have learned by offering an activity that you know interests her.

If a woman is interested in you and is open to going out, offering a date involving one of her favorite activities is not that important. Any date that sounds safe and comfortable will probably be accepted. If a woman has not decided whether she wants to go out with you, however, the activity that you suggest can be critical. Suggest an unappealing activity and you might get a rejection. Suggest an activity that she likes and she might be interested enough to accept.

In order to get a date with Rita, Larry had to suggest an activity that appealed to her. When they first met (in a health club), the conversation went something like this:

LARRY (*on an exercise machine next to Rita*): "Have you been a member of the club very long?"

RITA: "No. I'm new."

LARRY: "Did you belong to another club before?"

RITA: "No."

Their conversation continued like this for a few minutes, with Rita giving brief answers and showing little interest. Larry wanted to ask her out, and when she started getting off the exercise machine, he knew he had to do something fast.

LARRY: "Have you ever played racquetball?"

RITA (*finally showing some interest*): "No, but it looks like fun."

LARRY: "Want to have a game sometime? I'm not a great player, but I know enough to teach you how to play."

RITA (*after some hesitation*): "That would be okay."

LARRY: "Let's plan on next week. I'll call about a court. If you'll give me your number, I'll call you tomorrow and let you know what times are available."

Larry called Rita the next day, and they hit it off so well on the phone that they ended up going to dinner that evening. That was six months ago, and they are still seeing each other. Rita apologized to Larry for being so unfriendly when they first met. She said, "When I first met you I had just gone through a terrible divorce and I wasn't sure I was ready to start dating. Your offer to teach me how to play racquetball sounded like fun. It helped me make up my mind to get out and start living again."

Approaching a woman, carrying on a conversation, and asking for a date are not the easiest things in the world to do. If you get all the way to the point where you are going to ask for a date, don't jeopardize your chances of success by offering the *wrong* date. Offer a date that will give you the best chance of success—one she will feel is safe, comfortable, and enjoyable.

3

How to Turn
a No Into a Yes:
An Advanced Technique

When you ask a woman for a date but get turned down, how do you feel? If you are like most of us, you feel embarrassed, hurt, and maybe a little angry. In addition, you probably assume that she doesn't like you and doesn't want to go out with you. That's not necessarily so, however. Sometimes you will be turned down for a reason that has nothing to do with you. In that case, if you keep a cool head and analyze what's going on, you still might be successful. Here are four rules to follow when you get turned down.

FOUR RULES FOR TURNING A NO INTO A YES

Rule 1—Control Your Emotions

After dancing with a young lady, a cowboy in a western bar escorted her back to the table where her girlfriends were waiting. He then asked her if she would like to go out Saturday night. When she said she was busy, the cowboy turned and walked away, tipping up the back of his hat with his middle finger.

When most men ask for a date and get turned down, they stop thinking rationally and let their emotions take over. On rare occasions a man might do or say something offensive, as the cowboy in the above story did when he gave that young woman the single-finger salute. Most men, however, will simply end the conversation and go off to lick their wounds.

Even though your feelings may be hurt when you get turned down, don't assume that you have been rejected. Try to keep a clear head, because this is a critical moment. If you stay in control of your emotions, you might be able to turn the situation around.

Rule 2—Decide If You Got a Mixed Message

You have gotten a *mixed message* when a woman refuses your offer to go out, but:

1. She was talkative and friendly toward you before you asked for a date.
2. She gave an indefinite or tentative refusal such as, "Oh, I don't think I can."
3. She gave an excuse for not going out that could be either a gentle way of turning you down or the truth, such as, "I'm sorry, I'm busy that night."

On the other hand, you have gotten a *clear message* (i.e., a clear rejection) when:

1. She was cold and uncommunicative before you asked for a date.
2. With little hesitation, she turned you down with a flat "no" or "no, thank you."

When she has made it clear that she is not interested in a date with you, it's probably not worth pursuing the matter further. When you get a mixed message, however, by all means go on to Rule 3.

Rule 3—Understand Her Motivation

When you get a mixed message, proceed as if she likes you but has some concern about going out. Her concern could be simple, such as she really is busy Friday night, or it could be more complex, such as a fear of being hurt in a relationship. Your job is to figure out what her concern is. Sometimes it will be made obvious by what she says when she turns you down. Other times you won't have a clue and will have to ask questions to gain insight. Here are examples of how you could ask questions that might help you to better understand her concerns:

Example A

"Could I call on you sometime?"

(After a short pause) "No, I don't think so."

"Oh. Are you involved with someone?"

Example B

"Would you like to go to dinner Saturday night?"

"No, I just came out of a relationship. I'm not ready to start dating."

"That can be a tough time. How long since it ended?"

Example C

"Could we meet for lunch next week?"

"No, I'm awfully busy, but thank you for asking."

"Is your job keeping you busy?"

After gaining insight into her concerns, you may decide that she really doesn't like you, in which case you would be better off spending your time looking for someone else. If you decide that her refusal reflects a concern unrelated to you, however, proceed to Rule 4.

Rule 4—Offer a Revised Date

Once she has turned you down, you probably won't improve your chances by begging or getting pushy. To have the best chance of success, offer a revised date that addresses her concerns. Perhaps your offer needs to be for a safer date, a more casual date, a date at another time, or any revised date that you think will address her concerns.

Let's analyze a true story to see if following these four rules could have helped Denny get a date with Joyce. Here is Denny's story:

> Last year a woman was bludgeoned to death in her bed. The police said the killer had used a blunt instrument—possibly a hammer. The newspapers referred to the killer as "The Hammer Man." He was never caught.
>
> Two months after this murder I met a woman named Joyce at a singles dance. Joyce was just getting out on the singles scene after breaking up with her husband. She had brought her married sister to the dance to sort of act as a chaperon.
>
> Joyce and I hit it off right away. She was rubbing my back and snuggling up real close as we danced. After dancing and talking with Joyce for half an hour, I asked her if she would like to go out dancing sometime. She replied with a big smile, "Oh yes! *Anytime!*"
>
> We danced one more number and then took a break. Joyce disappeared into the rest room with her sister. When she returned, I tried to firm up our date, but something was wrong. Joyce wasn't smiling anymore and she was no longer willing to go on a date dancing with me. I could tell she was bothered by something. Suddenly she looked up at me and said, "Are you the Hammer Man?" I protested that I wasn't, but it didn't help— she still wouldn't agree to go out dancing. Her sister must have said something in the rest room that made her afraid. I was really frustrated because I liked her a lot and felt that she liked me. I was pretty upset. I left the dance without saying good-bye.

Let's see how Denny could have used the four rules to turn Joyce's no into a yes. When Joyce's eager acceptance of a date turned into a refusal, Denny got miffed and left the dance, killing any chance he had with her. He had clearly violated Rule 1 (Control Your Emotions). If he had kept his cool and proceeded to Rule 2 (Decide if You Got a Mixed Message), he would have realized that this was a classic case of getting a mixed message. After all, one minute Joyce was rubbing his back and saying that she would go out on a dancing date with him *anytime*, and then, a few minutes later, she was evasive about making a date. Recognizing that despite her refusal to go out, Joyce seemed to like him a lot, Denny could have gone on to Rule 3 (Understand Her Motivation) and explored her concerns. He didn't really need to ask Joyce any questions to understand her motivation, however, because her comment about the Hammer Man made it obvious that her problem was fear. Knowing this, Denny could have followed Rule 4 (Offer a Revised Date) and offered the safest date he could imagine. A suggestion that they meet for lunch would have been good, and to make it even safer he could have suggested making it a double date with her sister and brother-in-law. Such an offer might have made the difference. It certainly would have had a better chance for success than getting upset and leaving the dance.

APPLYING THE FOUR RULES

In the following situations, think for a moment about how you would apply the four rules for turning a no into a yes:

♦ You have been talking to a woman at a sidewalk café. She has been fun to talk to, so you ask her to meet you for lunch. She replies, "I'm sorry, I don't date."

♦ You have been talking to a woman at a singles dance. She seems to be enjoying your company, so you ask her to go out to dinner and a movie. She replies, "I'm sorry, I can't go. I'm married."

♦ You have been dancing with a woman in a singles bar. As you walk her back to her table, you ask her if she would like to go dancing sometime. She replies, "I'm sorry, I never date men I meet in bars."

If you received any of these answers, you might think that the refusal presented an insurmountable obstacle, or you might assume that the woman didn't like you and was just making up an excuse. Each of these replies, however, is really a statement about the woman herself, not you. We picked these three examples because in each case we have a true story about how a man was able to turn the no into a yes.

Let's take a look at what each man did. Here is what Dallas did when he met Linda in an outdoor café:

"I'm Sorry, I Don't Date"

Linda and I were seated near one another at an outdoor café and had gotten into an interesting conversation. After talking with her for about twenty minutes, I asked her out. The conversation went like this:

DALLAS: "Could we meet for lunch some day next week?"

LINDA: "I'm sorry, I don't date."

DALLAS: "And why is that?"

LINDA: "A year after my husband died I got involved with a man. We dated a year and he dropped me. I didn't need that after what I went through with my husband's death. Then I went out with a few other men and had a miserable time. I couldn't wait for the dates to end so I could get home. Finally, I just decided to avoid the whole hassle, so now I don't date. I am home alone a lot, though—it can get pretty lonely."

DALLAS: "Do you think you will ever remarry?"

LINDA: "Oh yes! I'll definitely remarry someday."

DALLAS (joking): "Who knows what the future holds. We might even get married someday, but don't you think we ought to have a date first? I'll tell you what, why don't we meet downtown at the Temple Hotel on Friday and do a little dancing? They have a live band. It should be fun. And since we can meet there, it won't really be a date. It will only be a half a date. Would you be up for that?"

LINDA: "I guess that would be OK. I can meet you there."

We traded numbers, and when I called to confirm the date, Linda said I could pick her up at her house.

When Linda said she didn't date, Dallas didn't get angry, nor did he pout and feel sorry for himself (Rule 1—Control Your Emotions). Because she seemed to enjoy his company, and because her reason for not going out was that she had decided not to date, Dallas realized that her refusal had nothing to do with him personally (Rule 2—Decide If You Got a Mixed Message). Dallas asked a question to find out why she didn't date (Rule 3—Understand Her Motivation). Her response to his question indicated that she was interested in having a man in her life, but was afraid of being hurt. He offered what he called a half-a-date, hoping that it would seem informal enough to be nonthreatening. Calling it a "half-a-date" also enabled her to accept his offer without going back on her statement that she didn't date (Rule 4—Offer a Revised Date).

Next is Byron's story:

"I'm Sorry, I Can't Go. I'm Married"

I met Donna at a singles dance I used to go to every Friday night. I found her very attractive and knew I wanted to go out with her. This is how our conversation went when I asked her for a date:

BYRON: "Would you like to go to dinner and a movie tomorrow night?"

DONNA: "I'm sorry, I can't go out with you. I'm married."

BYRON: "Does your husband care if you go out and dance with other men like this?"

DONNA: "He doesn't know where I am. Besides, we're getting divorced."

BYRON: "Are you separated?"

DONNA: "No. We're still living together because money is tight. But our divorce should be final in three weeks. He promised to move out by then."

BYRON: "Did you want the divorce?"

DONNA: "No, it's my husband's idea. He is much older than me, and he's leaving me for a younger woman. That's been pretty hard on my ego."

BYRON: "I've been through something like that myself and had a hard time of it. Do you think that perhaps we could meet for lunch? Sometimes it helps to talk these things over."

DONNA: "I really don't want to date until this is over. I have him in a box—he's giving me everything I want. I don't want to take the chance of messing up the agreement by getting him upset. But if you like we could meet here again next Friday. I would like to dance with you again."

When Donna turned down his offer of dinner and a movie, Byron just kept the conversation going as if nothing had happened (Rule 1—Control Your Emotions). She seemed to be having a good time dancing and talking with him, and her refusal to go out had nothing to do with him personally (Rule 2—Decide If You Got a Mixed Message), so he decided to ask her some questions about her situation (Rule 3—Understand Her Motivation). It didn't make sense that a married woman would be at a singles dance, so he asked her questions about her marriage. Her answers convinced him that what she really meant was she couldn't go out quite yet, and that was a whole different ball game. He thought that something less formal than the dinner date he had initially suggested might be acceptable, so he asked her if they could meet for lunch (Rule 4—Offer a Revised Date), but even that was unacceptable. When Donna suggested meeting at the dance the next Friday, however, the seemingly impossible situation of "I can't go out, I'm married" suddenly turned into a chance to see her again.

Here is Mike's experience in a singles bar:

"I'm Sorry, I Never Date Men I Meet in Bars"

I had been having a good time dancing and talking to Kathy. All the signs were positive. She smiled, talked freely, and appeared to be enjoying my company. After about fifteen minutes of dancing, the disc jockey stopped the music and announced there was going to be a name-that-tune contest. I decided to ask Kathy for a date as I walked her back to her table.

MIKE: "Would you like to go out dancing sometime?"

KATHY: "I'm sorry, I never date men I meet in bars, but we can dance again later."

MIKE "And why won't you date a man you met in a bar?"

KATHY: "I've just heard too many bad stories."

MIKE: "I know what you mean. I tell you what—here's my card. When you are going to come here dancing, would you give me a call? I'll meet you here and we can dance."

KATHY: "Okay, I'll take your card, but I want you to know, I never call men, so I probably won't call you."

At that point I walked Kathy back to her table and left her for a while. Later I went back and asked her to dance again. Once again she showed all the signs of liking me and having fun, and once again I tried for a date. Knowing Kathy had something against dating men she meets in a bar, I offered what I thought was a very safe date.

MIKE: "You know, I was just thinking, instead of going out dancing, could we meet for lunch next week?"

KATHY: "I'm sorry. It's a rule that I follow. I really never date a man I meet in a bar. But I have enjoyed dancing with you. Thank you very much."

Again I walked Kathy back to her table and went off to figure out my next move. Kathy seemed to enjoy my company, but she really seemed to have her mind made up about going out. The situation seemed pretty hopeless. However, when I was getting ready to leave for the evening, I decided to give it one last shot. I walked over to Kathy, and, as I was putting on my coat, had this conversation with her:

MIKE (joking): "Kathy, I'm going home now to wait for your call."

KATHY: "I probably won't call."

MIKE: "Is there absolutely positively no way we could meet? Perhaps we could meet at church?"

KATHY (*after a short pause*): "Okay you can call me at work. I'll give you my number. We can get together for lunch."

When we met for lunch Kathy said to me, "Do you know what you said that made me decide to go out with you? It was when you said we could meet at church. I figured that any man willing to meet at church had to be all right."

To get a date with Kathy, Mike had to be extremely patient. Not many men would still be smiling after so many rejections (Rule 1—Control Your Emotions). Because Kathy seemed to be enjoying his company and having a good time dancing with him, however, Mike felt that her refusal to go out only reflected her general concern about meeting a man in a bar and had nothing to do with him personally (Rule 2—Decide If You Got a Mixed Message). He did inquire about why she wouldn't date a man she met in a bar (Rule 3—Understand Her Motivation), but didn't learn much more from her vague answer, "I've just heard too many bad stories." When he offered to meet her for lunch (Rule 4—Offer a Revised Date) he got a second refusal, but he still kept his sense of humor (Rule 1—Control Your Emotions). Half jokingly, he offered to meet her at church. Kathy obviously wanted to go out with him, and his offer of a church meeting gave her the little nudge she needed to accept a lunch date.

You won't be able to turn every refusal into a date by applying these rules, not by a long shot. If the woman has been cold, does not seem to enjoy your company, and turns you down with a flat "no," your chances of getting a date are probably slim no matter what you do. But when she gives you a mixed message, you might be able to turn her no into a yes.

4

Where to Go

*a*fter a class in which we mention two dozen places to go, students often comment: "Tell us more places to go. You didn't tell us enough places." What they're really saying is, "Tell me an 'ideal' place to go where I will be comfortable, face no fear, experience no rejection, and end up meeting, and going out with, a desirable, attractive, quality person."

No wonder they want more places. None of the places we mention come close to this "ideal" place. Our places all require effort, facing fear, and braving possible rejection. We don't know of any ideal place. Granted, you may find some places easier, better, or more comfortable than others, but none we know of match this much-sought-after ideal place. Any given place will have a combination of characteristics that makes it closer to, or further from, the ideal.

The kind of place that best suits you, or any other person, is highly subjective. One person swears by watching a sports team, another loves the dance bars. One is sold on a singles sailing club while another says the shopping malls are the only way to go. No one place is perfect for everyone. Just because someone thinks a square dance club is a great place to meet someone doesn't necessarily mean it's right for you.

Although there is probably no perfect place for you, some may come closer to meeting your needs than others. Here are three questions to consider when deciding which places will suit you the best:

1. Is the place for singles or nonsingles?
2. Will the ratio be favorable?
3. Will compatible people be there?

IS THE PLACE FOR SINGLES OR NONSINGLES?

Singles places include activities, events, and organizations where the majority of those present are single people hoping to meet someone. Singles bars, social mixers, special singles events, and singles clubs are all included in the singles scenes category.

Nonsingles places include any place, activity, class, or organization that has a variety of people, most of whom are not single and are not there hoping to meet someone. Examples of the nonsingles places are work, shopping malls, city streets, parks, baseball games, office buildings, libraries, stores, restaurants, and organizations that don't cater to singles.

Some activities and organizations fall between the singles and nonsingles categories. A folk dance club may have many single members hoping to meet someone, while other members will be married or attached. Although singles places have advantages, so do nonsingles places. Let's take a look at the advantages of each.

Advantages of Singles Places

Many people, especially those recently single, are more comfortable meeting in places oriented to singles because most of those present will be unattached and open to meeting someone. It's not a surprise to anyone at a singles place if you approach a woman, talk to her, and ask for a date. This is expected and considered normal. If you are in a conversation with a woman at a singles event, you can be fairly sure her husband won't show up and wonder what you're up to. You can't be so sure of this in a nonsingles place. If you approach a woman in a shopping mall, her husband might be nearby.

Advantages of Nonsingles Places

Those who have experience trying to meet women often recognize a significant advantage of nonsingles places. That is, it's often easier to meet attractive women in a nonsingles place than in a singles place.

Here's why. The woman you meet in a nonsingles place is probably exposed to fewer meeting opportunities than the woman you meet in a singles place. The woman in a nonsingles place may not go to single events, may not have many opportunities for dates, and therefore may be more open to meeting you. A woman you meet at a singles place, by contrast, probably has many dating opportunities causing her to be more selective and possibly less interested in you.

Buddy, a friend of ours, told us how he benefited from this non-singles advantage.

It was Saturday morning. I had been out until 2:00 A.M. the night before, getting rejected by a multitude of women. Looking out the balcony of my condo, I saw this very attractive bikini-clad young woman sunbathing by the pool. She was definitely good-looking, and I wanted to meet her. After struggling to work up my courage, I went down to the pool.

Feeling conspicuous, I sat beside her and said, "Is it warm enough for you today?" Without smiling she said, "Yes, it is," and continued reading her book. After a few tense minutes I tried again. "Have you lived here long?" She answered and asked me how long I'd lived there. As our conversation continued, she began to relax and smile. When she got up to leave, I asked her to go to dinner. She seemed uncertain and said, "Well, I'm not sure. I would have to get a sitter." I said that would be fine, and I offered to pay for the sitter. She agreed and we arranged the details.

As I later found out, she had come from a small town, was recently divorced, and was uncomfortable meeting men and going out on dates. She was better looking than any of the women who had rejected me in the clubs the night before. If she had been in the clubs, lots of men would have been after her, and I don't think I would have had a chance.

Buddy took a chance in a nonsingles environment, and it paid off. He met someone at the pool whom he probably couldn't have met in a singles spot.

Another advantage of nonsingles places is that they lack the dreaded meat-market atmosphere associated with singles places. As a student of ours explained, "All the books I have read for singles focus on going to singles functions. The opportunities of meeting in nonsingles places are never mentioned. I dislike the meat-market feeling of singles places, and I am not very successful there. I find the nonsingles activities more interesting and, in many ways, a more romantic way to meet somebody."

Don't limit your choices. Consider both singles and nonsingles places when you are deciding where to go.

WILL THE RATIO BE FAVORABLE?

How important is the ratio of men to women at a given place or activity? Greg, a student in one of our classes who had limited meeting skills, thought it was very important, so important he went to the trouble of finding an organization with an amazingly good ratio. Here is what he told our class.

> I work for a large company which has a club to promote women as managers. Since the club is open to men as well as women, I joined. There were three men and ninety-two women. I've been to three meetings and have gotten a lot of attention.

Greg gets an A for originality. He certainly doesn't have to worry about competition in that environment. It makes sense: everything else being equal, the better the ratio, the better for you. But everything else *isn't* always equal. Ron, a friend of ours who likes to dance, explains.

> I never pay attention to the number of men in a dance spot compared to the number of women. Most of the men are just standing there doing nothing or talking to their friends. They are not actively trying to meet women and offer me no competition. The ratio in dance spots doesn't matter to me.

How skilled you are at the Five Steps determines how important the ratio is to you. If you are not very skilled, a good ratio is more important. If, however, you are adept at using the Five Steps, a good ratio is not critical.

Tip: Sometimes it is easy to find out what the ratio is. For instance, if you're considering taking an adult enrichment class, call the school and ask how many men and women are signed up for the class. Many schools will give you this information.

WILL COMPATIBLE PEOPLE BE THERE?

Many compatibility characteristics have obvious connections with places to go. If you want to meet a woman of a certain religion, attend church and church-related activities. If you like to garden, try a gardening club, lectures on gardening, or the gardening section of a bookstore. Like to sail? Try a sailing club. Given your requirements and some thought, you can often find a surprising number of places to find compatible women.

In Chapter 1, we showed you how Jim filled out the form "The Type of Woman I Want to Meet." Jim wanted an outdoor-loving woman who was free to travel on the weekends. Jim then used his requirements to determine places to go where he would have a good chance of meeting a compatible woman, as his "Where I Will Go" form shows (see page 51).

A blank "Where I Will Go" form, is included in Appendix A. Here is what Jim said after he filled out his list:

Going through the "Where I Will Go" list made me realize that each place had pluses and minuses. Group hikes, for example, are very appealing because women who hike are likely to enjoy the active outdoor life I enjoy. That's the advantage of group hikes. The downside of meeting someone hiking is that the hikes are only available during summer weekends.

So I ended up with a variety of places. Some of them, like hiking, depend on the season. Others, like slide shows and lectures on travel, are independent of the season and go on year round. I also go to places like dance bars that don't have a high proportion of compatible women. The advantage of a dance bar is its availability. It is open almost every night of the year. If I have nothing better to do, I will go there.

It didn't take Bill, a rocket scientist friend of ours, long to determine the best place for him.

I found myself divorced after many years of marriage and, by fate, found a fairly easy method for meeting women. Before our divorce, my wife and I belonged to a local folk dance club. After my divorce, I continued folk dancing. It kept me busy doing an activity I enjoyed and put me in contact with many quality single women. There would invariably be more women than men at the dances. They were easy to meet—just ask them to dance. And there was definitely no meat-market atmosphere since over half of the dancers were married or involved.

I also like to bike, and one time I went on a singles bike ride sponsored by a conservation group. There were ten men and three women. It didn't take a rocket scientist to figure out that folk dancing was a better way for me to spend my time. I am now married, and as you might guess, I met her folk dancing.

Bill used his folk dancing interest as an easy way to meet compatible women in a nonsingles environment that had more women than men. Not a bad combination.

It will probably take you some time to determine the best places for you. Although no one place is likely to be easy, some will be easier and more productive for you than others. The places you go will likely change as you gain experience and find out what works and what doesn't. Start by filling out the forms in Appendix A: "The Type of Woman I Want to Meet" and "Where I Will Go." Also look through Appendix D, "A Sampling of Places to Go and Things to Do," which lists activities we found in an entertainment weekly newspaper, the entertainment section of a daily newspaper, an adult enrichment class catalog, and the yellow pages. Then spend some time, preferably with a friend, brainstorming about places you could go. Try out some of these places and evaluate your results.

Jim's Choices on the "Where I Will Go" Form

(Use Your Requirements as a Guide)
(Y = Yes, N = No, M = Maybe)

Places, Activities, & Organizations	Y	N	M
Adult enrichment classes			M
Aerobics classes			M
Amusement parks		N	
Apartment bldg. pools & rec rooms			M
Art museums			M
Ballroom dance clubs			M
Beaches			M
Bicycle group tours			M
Bicycling clubs			M
Bike paths	Y		
Block parties		N	
Book discussion groups		N	
Bookstores with reading areas			M
Botanical gardens		N	
Bowling leagues		N	
Bus tours		N	
Camping clubs			M
Charities		N	

Places, Activities, & Organizations	Y	N	M
Charity and fund-raising events		N	
City parks	Y		
City streets (busy areas)			M
Civic groups		N	
Coffeehouses for sitting and reading			M
Computer user groups		N	
Conservation organizations			M
Country and Western dance clubs			M
Country clubs		N	
Cross-country ski races			M
Cruises		N	
Dance spots	Y		
Dog owners and breeders clubs		N	
Dog shows		N	
Downtown celebrations			M
Environmental groups			M
Equestrian clubs		N	
Ethnic clubs		N	
Festivals (music, beer, seasonal, etc.)			M
Folk dancing clubs			M
Food courts			M

Places, Activities, & Organizations	Y	N	M
Foreign language clubs		N	
Gambling casinos		N	
Gardening clubs		N	
Golf courses		N	
Health clubs	Y		
Hiking	Y		
Historical museums		N	
Historical societies		N	
Homeowners associations		N	
Horse races		N	
Ice rinks			M
I.Q. clubs		N	
Lectures	Y		
Libraries			M
Motorcycle clubs		N	
Natural history museums		N	
Outdoor adventure tours			M
Outdoor clubs			M
Overweight singles clubs		N	
Parent organizations		N	
Parent/school organizations		N	

Places, Activities, & Organizations	Y	N	M
Parties			M
Playgrounds		N	
Poetry reading clubs		N	
Political organizations		N	
Professional clubs of various types		N	
Professional singles clubs		N	
Public speaking clubs		N	
Recreation centers	Y		
Recreational vehicle clubs		N	
Religious organizations		N	
Resorts		N	
Roller skating rinks		N	
Runs and triathalons	Y		
Sailing clubs		N	
Self-help and therapy groups		N	
Shopping malls			M
Singles bars			M
Single parents clubs		N	
Singles support groups		N	
Ski clubs			M
Ski resorts	Y		

Places, Activities, & Organizations	Y	N	M
Soccer clubs			M
Social mixers			M
Softball teams		N	
Swimming clubs		N	
Tall clubs		N	
Tennis clubs		N	
Theater groups		N	
Touch football teams		N	
Travel clubs			M
Volunteer organizations			M
Widows and widowers clubs		N	
Zoos		N	
Other:			
Other:			
Other:			
Other:			
Other:			
Other:			
Other:			
Other:			
Other:			

5

Success in a New Place in Three Easy Phases

*I*n our class, the question we are asked most frequently is, "Where's a good place to go to meet someone?" We respond by suggesting a variety of places. When we are discussing the merits of a place, however, a student will typically break in with, "That's not a good place to go. I went there once and didn't meet anybody. I'm not going back." The students who say this don't realize that it's unrealistic to expect success going to a place only one time. For most people, it takes a lot more than one visit to get comfortable in a new place and to figure out ways to meet someone there.

We have developed a three-phase system that makes it easier to become comfortable and effective at meeting women in a new place. This approach works in typical meeting places such as singles mixers and singles bars, and it also works in more unusual places to meet such as video stores and libraries. Here are the three phases:

PHASE 1—EXPLORE

On your first few visits, go with the intention of exploring the place, not with the intention of meeting someone. These first few visits are fact-finding trips. If you do happen to meet a woman right away, that's great, but don't count on it because it probably won't happen. Instead, the purpose of these early visits is to:

See Who Is There

How many women are there? Are they the right age? How many do you find appealing? If there is no one there you would want to meet, maybe you shouldn't return. Don't be too quick to judge, however. We have heard it many times—a friend or one of our students will go to an event where there are five hundred women and then say, "There wasn't anyone there I liked." We find that hard to believe. We suspect these men were reacting in a negative way because they were afraid of the new situation.

Become at Ease in the New Environment

If you are like most people, you have a tendency to keep to yourself when around strangers in a strange environment. As you become more at ease, however, you probably become more outgoing and find it easier to strike up conversations. To give yourself a chance to become at ease when trying a new place, go at least three times. We have seen many negative first impressions turn positive after a few subsequent visits. Allow more than three visits to get comfortable in singles bars, singles mixers, and other places that have a meat-market atmosphere.

Think of Ways to Apply the Five Steps

On your first few visits, whether it's to a singles dance or a shopping mall, you probably won't know how to make contact. But there's a way to learn. While you are spending time getting comfortable in a new place, think of ways to apply each of the Five Steps in that environment. After you analyze each step, what at first seemed impossible might become quite doable.

PHASE 2—EXPERIMENT

After you have become somewhat at ease in a place and have thought of several ways to apply the Five Steps, start experimenting. Try one way of doing the Five Steps, evaluate your results, modify your methods, and try again. It's a trial and error process. In this experimental phase you will be concentrating on how to get near, break the ice, and continue the conversation. The first step, searching, is usually not difficult, and the last step, closing, is not an issue until you have some success with the first four steps.

You might quickly arrive at an effective way to apply the Five Steps and decide to stick with that method, or you might experiment with different methods over a period of time before settling on one (or more) that works for you. Don't be discouraged if it takes a long time to get the hang of meeting women in any particular place. If you are there and trying, you are head and shoulders above those who are sitting at home waiting for their luck to change.

PHASE 3—EXECUTE

Typically, the experiment phase slowly evolves into the execute phase. As you gain experience, you will experiment less and less. Instead, you will use tried and true methods that you know will work. You may still be "fine tuning" your methods, but you won't be making big changes. When you get to the execute phase you will be able to easily meet and evaluate a variety of potential partners.

Reed, a student of ours, had some expertise meeting women in singles bars. He had no trouble asking women to dance, and, if he liked them, he had no trouble asking them out. In singles bars Reed had progressed to the execute phase. Even though he often went to singles bars, however, he hadn't ended up in a relationship. He thought a different meeting environment might help, and he asked us to suggest a new place. When we recommended a food court at a mall, Reed was noticeably troubled. Even though he could approach women with ease at a dance spot, we could tell the thought of approaching a woman in a food court made him uncomfortable. To give him confidence, we explained our three-phase system and gave him a pep talk. We also asked him to keep a record of his progress at the food court. Here's what he wrote:

REED'S FOOD COURT DIARY

Sunday, July 17

Today I made an exploratory visit to the food court. If I had been there just to eat, I would have been totally relaxed, but since I was there trying to learn how to meet women, I had butterflies in my stomach. Even though I had no intention of talking to any woman on this visit, I was still nervous.

I took a book to read so I wouldn't feel conspicuous hanging around a long time. I sat at a table for three hours reading and sipping coffee. Occasionally I would look around to see what kind of women were there and try to think of ways to approach them.

I noticed a lot of women were walking fast and carrying packages, obviously busy shopping. They looked as if they would be hard to approach. Other women were seated at tables talking to friends, as if they had the whole afternoon to kill. Some women were sitting alone having snacks. They looked as if they would be the easiest to meet. There were a lot of college age women, alone and in groups, probably from a nearby campus. Several women working behind the food counters were appealing. This visit convinced me that the food court has a lot of potential as a place to meet women.

There are several ways I could apply the Five Steps. The search step should be easy. I could either walk around the court to see who is there or keep an eye open while seated. I thought of four ways to get near and break the ice:

1. If a woman is standing in line at a food counter, I could stand next to her, talk to her briefly, and then ask if she would like to join me for some conversation while we eat.
2. I could walk up to a woman seated at a table and ask her if she would like some conversation while she eats, and then sit at her table if she says it's okay.
3. If a woman is sitting at a table, I could sit at an adjacent table and start a conversation from there. If the conversation goes well, I could move over to her table.

4. If a woman working behind a counter isn't busy, I could get a conversation going with her.

At the end of the three hours I felt more at home at the food court. The thought of approaching a woman there is becoming a little less frightening.

Reed was in the explore phase on his Sunday afternoon visit. He spent a good deal of time at the food court, which helped him feel more relaxed in that environment, and he observed what type of women were there and what they were doing, all exploratory activities. He also came up with several ways to search, get near, and break the ice. Let's see what he did on his second visit.

Tuesday, July 19
Tonight I had a late dinner at the food court after my night school class. My goal was to experiment with ways to make contact. Even though I was only going to "experiment," I had to work hard to get my nerve up. I still had butterflies in my stomach.

While I was walking around in "search mode," I noticed a woman waiting in line to get Greek food. I got in line behind her and said, "What looks good to you?" She gave me a friendly response, and we started talking about the food. After a couple of minutes, even though I was scared to death, I said, "Are you with anyone? Would you like to eat together?" She pointed to a man at a table and said, "I'm with my uncle." When I saw him I knew I wasn't going to take this any further. Her uncle (if that's who he really was) was a big, tough-looking guy. He was watching us and he wasn't smiling.

Even though my first attempt at meeting a woman at the food court failed, I felt good about myself. At least I hadn't chickened out.

After I got my Greek dinner I looked around for a woman eating alone. I didn't see anyone I wanted to meet, so I picked a table where I could watch women walk by. Several appealing women did walk by, but I couldn't figure out any way to get them to stop so I could talk to them.

After eating, I saw a cute woman standing at the cookie counter. I quickly went over to buy a cookie. The salesgirl told me they were about to close, so it was two cookies for the price of one. I offered the extra cookie to the woman I wanted to meet (she was still trying to decide what to buy). She took the cookie and said, "Why, thank you." She stood there a couple of seconds. I got tongue-tied and didn't know what else to say. She walked away. One more failure, but at least I did a couple of the steps.

I looked around for a place to eat my cookie and spotted a woman who was sitting alone looking bored. I thought that was a good sign—it might mean she was open to some company. I sat at an adjacent table, made eye contact, and said, "If you hurry, you can get twofers at the cookie stand." She smiled and said, "I just had an ice cream. I'd better let it go at that." We continued chatting for a few minutes. Even though I didn't find her appealing after talking to her, I was encouraged by how easy it was to strike up a conversation with someone seated at a nearby table.

Sitting near a woman might be the best way for me to get near and start a conversation. This seems better than talking to a woman while standing because I can avoid the awkward moment when I have to ask if I can sit with her. In addition, if I am seated near a woman and can't think of anything to say for a moment, the conversation won't necessarily end. I can just sit there until something comes to mind. Even though I had no success getting a date tonight, I am getting excited about the possibilities.

On his second visit, Reed progressed to the experimental phase. He tried several ways to get near and break the ice. He got in line behind a woman at the Greek food stand, offered a cookie to a woman at the cookie concession, and talked to another woman while seated at a table. He was figuring out ways to apply the Five Steps at a food court.

Thursday, July 21
Today I stopped at the food court for dinner after work. I decided to use the method where I would sit near someone I

wanted to meet. While I was standing with my tray looking around for a woman to sit near, I saw an attractive woman on the other side of the court. She put her tray on a table and then left for a moment. While she was gone, I took a seat at the table next to hers. I picked a chair where I would be close enough to speak. When she returned she was carrying a singles newspaper opened to an ad for Jinks (a local dance spot). As she sat down, she looked at me and said, "Do you know where this place is? I would like to see what it's like."

I slid out of my chair and into a chair at her table so I could read the ad. I told her how to get to Jinks and then introduced myself. Her name was Danna. We continued talking for half an hour. When Danna said, "I'm new in town and don't know many people," I felt she was hinting that she wanted me to ask her out. I had intended to anyway—this just made it easier. I said, "Would you like to see the downtown sights with me Saturday night? We could get a bite to eat and then hit some of the dance spots." Danna agreed, and suggested we start with Jinks.

Reed never progressed to Phase 3 where he knew without a doubt what would work best for him in a food court. When he met Danna he was still in Phase 2, experimenting with ways to apply the Five Steps.

When you try a new place, you might progress as rapidly as Reed, or you might take longer to feel sufficiently at ease to experiment with ways to apply the Five Steps. Reed's experience in singles bars probably helped him make rapid progress at the food court.

Whether you want to try a new place to see some new faces or you are new to the singles scene and every place you try is new, this three-phase approach will help you become more successful. Even if you've already used the recommendations in Chapter 4 to choose places which give you a better chance of success, applying this three-phase approach as well will be useful. The way we look at it, no matter what the place or event is, if there are appealing women there, they can be met. It's only a matter of learning how.

How to Meet Women in Your Daily Life

You are in a shopping mall when you see an appealing woman who is alone and not wearing a wedding ring. You would love to meet her, so what do you do? If you are like most men, you do nothing at all. Perhaps you try to console yourself and your lack of nerve by thinking, "She probably wouldn't want to go out with me anyway." This thought is more of an excuse than a reflection of reality. Until you ask a woman for a date, you really don't know if she would go out with you. Since you didn't ask, you have passed up an opportunity.

You don't have to keep missing these opportunities. Here are some fairly simple habits you can develop that will dramatically improve your chances of meeting a woman while you are going about your routine daily activities.

HABIT NO. 1—ACTIVELY LOOK FOR MEETING OPPORTUNITIES.

Don't be in a fog as you go about your daily tasks, unaware of the many meeting opportunities that are around you. Wherever you are, be aware of the possibilities. Jim, a friend of ours, actively looks for opportunities to meet a woman—even when he is at the gas station:

> Whenever I drive into a gas station, I always look to see who is at the pumps. If there is a woman pumping gas, I pull up to the pump nearest her. If I can't think of anything better to say, I start a conversation by saying, "What kind of mileage does your car get?" Most of the time we just have a short conversation, but occasionally there's more. One time I noticed a woman getting out of her car who was all dressed up. I pulled up to the nearest pump, and as I got out of my car, I said, "You don't look like you're dressed for pumping gas; could I do that for you?" She accepted my offer, and we talked while I filled her tank. We hit it off, and after a short conversation, I made a date to take her to lunch that very day.

Bruce is another friend who stays alert for opportunities to meet women. He kept his eyes open one day in a store, recognized an opportunity, and took advantage of it. Here is what he told us.

> When I was in a discount store shopping for a cordless phone, an appealing saleswoman waited on me. She wasn't wearing a wedding ring, and she seemed very nice. I wanted to get a date with her, but I had never asked out a saleswoman in a store before, so I wasn't sure how to go about it.
>
> I started by asking questions about the cordless phones. The store didn't have the one I was looking for, so I soon ran out of questions. I was right on the verge of thanking her and moving on (I was getting pretty nervous), but I mustered up the nerve to ask her some personal questions. I asked Donna (she had a name tag on) how she had gotten into sales. She said that she had a degree in psychology, and sales was dealing with people, so it wasn't too much of a mismatch. She said she also worked nights as an improvisational comedian. I kept the conversation going a couple of minutes more by asking her where she worked as a comedian and what it was like being on stage. However, I

knew I couldn't keep this conversation up very long because there was another customer waiting at the end of the counter, so I just came right out and asked her if she would like to go to dinner sometime. She got completely flustered and said, "I don't know what to say. This has never happened to me before." Without giving me a yes or no, Donna said that she had to take care of the customer who was waiting, but would be back.

Her reaction was interesting. She was very attractive, so I figured that men must have been asking her out all day long, but apparently not. When she had finished with the customer, I said, "Have you had time to think about going to dinner with me?" She replied, "I will go if we can meet somewhere rather than you picking me up." That sounded reasonable to me, so we arranged to meet for dinner and traded phone numbers.

Do you actively look for meeting opportunities as you go about your daily tasks? If you do, you are less likely to be caught off guard when an opportunity suddenly presents itself. Don't get so wrapped up in the errand you are running that you fail to recognize that you are close to, looking at, or talking to, a potential romantic partner.

Habit No. 2—Plan the Five Steps

One way to ensure that you will take some action is to plan the Five Steps before you need to use them. Planning prepares you for action. On your way to a store, the bank, the post office, or anyplace else where there might be women, plan how you will apply the Five Steps at that place. When you arrive, put your plan into action, starting with the search. Searching will put you in an active mode and make you more likely to proceed with the other steps. Since you will be meeting the woman in a nonsingles situation, pay special attention to the two conversation goals of getting insurance and extending your time together.

Frank, an acquaintance of ours in his early sixties, takes advantage of meeting opportunities that arise in some unusual places, such as (would you believe) a hardware store. Every time he goes there, he has a little plan that he executes. Here is what he told us about his hardware store strategy:

> On the way to the hardware store one day, I gave some thought to how to meet a woman there. I came up with a plan, and it seems to work. The way I see it, any woman alone in a hardware store probably doesn't have a man in her life, and it's quite likely that she has a problem with her house that she's trying to fix. It's also quite likely she would like some help fixing that problem. So when I get to the hardware store, I do a little search to see if there is an appealing woman there alone. If there is, I just go up to her and say, "And what broke this time?" When she tells me what her problem is, I analyze it, help her find what she needs, and give her advice on how to make the repair. Women are almost always appreciative. If there seems to be some chemistry, I'll ask her out.

Before Frank had a plan, he would walk into the hardware store, get what he needed, and leave. Now when he goes to the hardware store, he sometimes gets what he *really* wants—a date with an appealing woman.

HABIT NO. 3—VARY WHEN AND WHERE YOU GO

If your daily routine takes you to the same places at the same time every day, you will be exposed to pretty much the same people day after day. By varying the time or place, you will see more new faces. For example, if you eat lunch at eleven-thirty every day, try eating at twelve thirty some days, or eat in a different place. If your daily workout is at noon, vary your routine and occasionally go after work. If you eat breakfast at home every day, eat in a restaurant once in a while. If you normally drive to work, try the bus.

All Randy did was change the place he ate lunch—it paid off.

> Before I got divorced, my lunchtime routine was pretty set. I would work out for an hour and then eat lunch in my office. One

day, several months after my divorce, I made a conscious decision to change my routine and eat lunch in the main company cafeteria. I wanted to see if there were any women there who interested me. After I got my tray, I looked around and noticed two women sitting with an empty table next to them, so I sat at that table. Overhearing their conversation, I learned that the one without a wedding ring was the owner of an art gallery, and she was exhibiting wildlife paintings in the cafeteria lobby. I started a conversation with her by saying, "Are those your paintings in the lobby?" We talked about her gallery, and eventually I asked for her business card. That afternoon I called her and invited her to join me for dinner. We've been together for two years now.

Randy made a change in his routine and got a quick payoff. He was certainly not going to meet a woman by having lunch in his office.

HABIT NO. 4—SPEAK TO STRANGERS

Do you have trouble striking up conversations with appealing women? Here is a painless way to get better. As you go about your daily tasks, practice striking up conversations with strangers. Don't limit your practice to just women who interest you. Practice on everyone—men, women, and children—and practice every chance you get. The more you practice on people you are not romantically interested in, the better prepared you will be when it comes time to speak to a woman who has a romantic appeal.

If you frequently go to any one place, such as a health club, supermarket, or mall, develop expertise at meeting women at that place. Because you go often, it will be worth your time to develop a plan for applying the Five Steps in that environment, and you will have plenty of opportunities to try your plan, analyze your results, modify your plan, and try it again.

Kevin spends a lot of time in the library studying. When he wants to meet a woman, he has a plan that he puts into action whenever he is there. Here is what he does:

I go to the library to study several times a week, so I have developed a method for meeting women there. Before I sit down, I look at all the long tables to see if there are any women sitting there with an empty seat near them. If so, I take the seat, get out my books and paper, and study for several minutes. Then I say something like, "You are studying hard tonight." Many times I get little response from the comment. The woman might be polite, but not interested in talking. But every once in a while a woman is eager to have someone to talk to. If, after several minutes of chatting, she still seems interested, I suggest taking a coffee break together. I have met a lot of women this way.

Kevin went to the library frequently, so he developed expertise in that situation. For him, it is a way to meet women that takes little extra time.

During one of our classes we asked the women to describe the boldest approach a man had ever used to meet them. Janet told us she had been at the shopping mall one evening, and a man came up to her and said, "Hi! My name is Chuck. I don't want to be rude, but I couldn't help noticing you. I wonder if you would go to dinner with me sometime?" The class seemed amazed at Chuck's approach. One man laughed at Janet's story and said, "How could he expect a woman to go out with a total stranger when he used an abrupt approach like that?" He stopped laughing, however, when we asked Janet how she responded, and she said, "I went out with him."

Many men try to make contact with women only when they are in "normal" meeting places, such as work, a singles bar, a party, or a singles mixer. Meeting in the normal places is fine, but don't forget about the possibilities you have as you go about your routine tasks. Make meeting women in your daily life part of your campaign to find the right woman.

7

Help for Single Dads

*a*ndre, a student in one of our classes, raised an important issue when he said, "I have two sons in grade school. I would like to meet a woman who has kids about the same age as my boys, but so far I haven't had any success. I have my boys on weekends so I don't get out Friday or Saturday night, and I don't get out much during the week because I have to get up so early for work. With my kind of schedule, how can I meet a single mother with young children?"

Andre has two problems: (1) he doesn't have much time to spend looking for a woman; and (2) he doesn't know where to go to find a woman who would be open to his children (that is, a woman who has young children of her own).

There is a way to solve the "no time to look" problem and the "how to meet someone with children" problem simultaneously. Make your time do double duty by looking for a woman while you are enjoying activities with your children. Get your kids away from the TV and take them places where there will be other children and their single mothers. Here are some suggestions for places to take your children:

Amusement parks	Children's museums
Beaches	Children's theater
Bike paths	Church activities
Campgrounds	City zoos
Children's concerts	Company picnics

Fairs	Petting zoos
Fun centers in malls, etc.	Restaurants with playlands, video games, or clowns
Hiking clubs with family activities	School activities
Libraries	Single-parent clubs with family activities
Museums	
Parks with playgrounds	Swimming pools

After reading this list, Jay, a single friend of ours, said, "The zoo? Go to the zoo to meet somebody? Is this some kind of a joke? You've got to be kidding!" We aren't kidding—far from it. If you want to meet a single mom, zoos, as well as the other places on the list, can be excellent places to go. Because these places aren't usually thought of as singles meeting places, however, few people there will be making a conscious effort to make contact. To have a good chance of meeting someone at such places you have to do more than just be there; you have to apply the Five Steps.

Being with your children can sometimes make executing the Five Steps easier than if you were alone. Hal found this out one day when he was at the beach with his son Gary. Even though Hal had spent a lot of time at the beach with Gary, he had not met one woman, until he came up with a unique approach.

When Gary was a little boy I used to take him to the beach on my visitation weekends. There were all kinds of women there, but for a long time I couldn't figure out how I could meet any of them. I just didn't have the nerve to walk right up to a woman and start talking. Then one day I noticed a woman lying on her towel near the water. Her son was close by, playing in the wet sand. Suddenly I had a stroke of genius—Gary could help me meet this woman.

I pointed the other boy out to Gary as I said, "Gary, look at that little boy over there playing all alone. Why don't you go help him build a sand castle?" Gary thought this was a great idea. He picked up his bucket and shovel and went over and started building a sand castle with the woman's son.

After a few minutes, I wandered over to examine the sand castle. Gary's new friend called out to his mom, "Mommy! Look at what we are making." I turned to her and said, "I think we have two civil engineers here." She laughed, and got up to take a closer look at what our "engineers" were building. Talking about the boys made it easy to keep the conversation going. I never really had a chance to get cold feet.

Hal had made his time at the beach do double duty. He was able to spend time with his son and also meet a woman. By having Gary play with the woman's son, he was able to get near, break the ice, and continue the conversation. Gary benefited by having a playmate.

Tip: *A park, as well as a beach, can be a great place to meet single mothers with young children, but not just any park. Some parks cater more to adults, with jogging paths and facilities such as tennis courts. Others cater more to young children and have swings, slides, and swimming pools. To find the parks with the greatest potential for meeting single moms who are out with their kids, locate the parks in your area on a city map and then try a different park on each outing.*

When you go to a singles function such as a singles bar, singles dance, or singles mixer, you might assume that most women there are unattached and interested in a relationship, and you would probably be right. You can likely make the same assumption when you see children accompanied by only their mother at a zoo, beach, or amusement park on a Saturday, Sunday, or holiday. Because these are "family" activities, there is an excellent chance that the mother is single and not involved with anyone. If she were involved with someone, the odds are that "someone" would be with her on such a family outing.

Tip: When you see a single mother exasperated with her children, consider it a meeting opportunity. Her frustration gives you a chance to break the ice by offering a sympathetic remark and maybe some help.

Be a good parent and spend time with your children. Be good to yourself and use this time to meet someone who can enhance your life. Your time can do double duty.

8

Spend Money Once—
Meet Women Forever

Some men are willing to spend a lot of money if they think it will help them find a mate. For example, a personal ad in a singles newspaper read, "Find a wife for lonely businessman and get $10,000." Some dating services charge thousands of dollars for a membership, but what happens if you are lucky enough to meet a woman through such a service, and later your membership and relationship both expire? What happens is you have to spend the money all over again.

There is another way to meet women that requires spending money only once, and for your money you get a guaranteed way to meet women for the rest of your life. We are talking about spending money on dance lessons. Knowing how to dance is a golden key to meeting women. If you already know how to dance, you know this is true. If you cannot dance, then take lessons, and join the ranks of the men who use this fun and easy way to meet women.

You don't have to be a highly skilled dancer to start meeting women. You can start meeting women as soon as you learn the basic steps. The better you get, however, the more advantages there are. Here are some of the advantages of being able to dance at different levels.

Beginner
(You know one or two basic steps and can lead easy turns.)

♦ You will be able to take advantage of the many places that have dancing. In addition to all the singles bars and singles dances, many social gatherings such as weddings and private parties have dancing.

♦ You will be able to meet women by using the icebreaker, "Would you like to dance?" This is an easy icebreaker to use because it's an accepted question wherever there is dancing, and it is not necessary to have any immediate follow-up conversation.

♦ On a dance floor you will have a woman all to yourself. She won't be dividing her attention between you and her girl-friend, and no other men will be likely to interrupt your conversation.

♦ When dancing, you will have the woman's hand in yours, and your faces and bodies will be close or touching. This intimate contact might get the chemistry started.

♦ If you are dancing with a woman and decide that you are not interested in her, it will be easy to end the conversation by walking her off the dance floor and thanking her for the dance. No awkward excuse for ending the conversation will be necessary.

Intermediate
(You can lead a woman fairly well in a variety of different dances.)
Being able to dance at the intermediate level has all the advantages listed for the beginner level, plus these additional advantages:

♦ You will seldom have to pass up a chance to ask a woman to dance because you can't dance to a certain type of music.

♦ You will seldom have to leave the dance floor because the music has changed to something you can't dance to.

- ◆ You will make your dance partner feel at ease on the dance floor. If she feels comfortable, she will be more likely to continue dancing with you. This will give the two of you more time to get acquainted.
- ◆ You will be comfortable asking a woman for a date to go dancing.

Advanced

(You can dance well to any music played. Your ability to lead is a delight to women because it makes them look good and feel good on the dance floor.)

Being able to dance at the advanced level has all the advantages listed for the beginner and intermediate levels, plus these additional advantages:

- ◆ Knowing that you are an excellent dancer may give you the confidence to ask beautiful women to dance and to go out on dancing dates.
- ◆ Your ability to dance will make more women want to go out with you.
- ◆ Some women have made dancing a central part of their lives and will not date men who are not good dancers. These women will be more available to you.

Rudy is a great dancer. There was a time when Rudy was embarrassed to be seen on the dance floor, but he took dance lessons and changed his life forever. Here is what he had to say about the benefits of being able to dance:

Years ago the only dance I could do was a slow shuffle in time with the music. When I saw a woman I wanted to meet, I had to wait for slow music before I could ask her for a dance. Even when slow music came on I had a hard time getting my nerve up to ask for a dance because I knew I wasn't a very good dancer. While I was waiting for the right music or waiting to get my nerve up, some other guy would usually ask her first;

then I would have to wait a long time before I would get another chance, if at all.

I got tired of seeing the good dancers get all the women, so I took dance lessons and practiced a lot. Now I have an entirely different attitude. I don't have to wait for slow music, and I won't hesitate to ask the best-looking lady in a place to dance, because I know if she accepts, I'm going to show her a good time on the dance floor.

Learning to dance has the potential to improve your love life more than almost anything else you can do. It worked for our friend Rudy, and it can work for you.

When we recommend that you learn to dance, we are talking specifically about learning the type of dancing where the man leads and the woman follows. We call this "touch" dancing. The fox-trot, waltz, and rumba are examples of touch dancing, as are the Texas two-step and three-step. Touch dancing is a great way to meet women because you have the woman in your arms where the two of you can easily talk and get to know one another.

"Freestyle" is a popular type of dancing where the man and woman dance apart without touching. Freestyle dancing, however, is of little use for meeting women. Because the music is so loud in the places that feature freestyle dancing and because you and your partner are dancing separately, it is extremely difficult to carry on a conversation. If you can't talk to your dance partner, you won't learn anything about her and she won't learn anything about you. You are no closer to getting a date after dancing with her than before. You would appear to be very abrupt if, after dancing with a woman, you were to ask her for a date without having had some conversation.

Tip: As far as meeting women goes, there is an even more useless type of dance than freestyle, and that is country-western line dancing. Line dances are done without a partner. Put these way down on your list of dances to learn.

When we recommend learning to dance to the men in our class, we get asked many questions about how to go about it. Here are some typical questions, and our answers:

WHICH DANCE SHOULD I LEARN FIRST?

You will have to choose between one of the country-western dances (the Texas two-step or three-step), a ballroom dance (the fox-trot or waltz), or a Latin dance (the cha-cha, tango, or rumba). Before you decide which dance to learn first, do some research to find dance spots in your area that will be good places to meet women. You are looking for places that are popular and plentiful in your metropolitan area and that feature touch dancing, attract the type of woman you are looking for, and draw large crowds (more women to choose from). Start by taking lessons in one of the dances that are popular at the clubs which appeal to you and seem to have a good potential for meeting women.

An easy way to do your research is to find just one dance spot and then ask the good dancers there where else they go to dance. Good dancers often explore a lot of different dance places, and they can tell you which of these places are good and which to avoid.

Another way to do your research is to look in entertainment weeklies, the entertainment section of your daily paper, or the yellow pages. Look in the yellow pages under such headings as "Bars," "Clubs," "Dancing," "Night Life," and any heading that starts with "Singles." In a large city there will be hundreds of places listed under some of these headings. Phone the places that give you some clue from their name that they might have dancing. Inquire whether they have dancing and if so, what type is most popular there. If a place features mostly touch dancing, inquire about the age of the clientele, the size of the crowds, and the best nights for meeting women.

When you are deciding where to go dancing to meet women, don't let your personal prejudices about music get in the way. In one of our classes we had just told the men about a country-western dance hall in town that draws about two thousand people on Friday and Saturday nights. We told the men, "That's a thousand women, most of whom are trying to meet a man." A man in the class said, "That place won't work for me. I don't like country music." We couldn't imagine such a reaction. We were teaching a class on how to meet women, not a music appreciation class.

SHOULD I TAKE GROUP OR PRIVATE LESSONS?

If you have plenty of money, the fastest way to learn to dance is to take private lessons. Group lessons are less expensive than private, but you might progress at a slower rate because group lessons are sometimes geared to the slowest member of the class. In a group lesson, however, you will get experience leading many different women, which can help you develop a good lead style. When you are taking private instructions from a woman instructor, you may get spoiled by how easy she is to lead. The women in a group class are more like the real world. If the cost is not prohibitive, consider a combination of group and private lessons as a way to learn quickly and to get practice leading a variety of women.

Another advantage to group lessons is that they provide an opportunity to meet single women during the lesson. Our friend Rudy got involved with a woman he met at a group country-western dance class. This is what happened:

A country-western bar that opened near my house offered free group dance lessons. I stopped in one night to check it out because I had been thinking about taking lessons. As soon as I walked in, I spotted a pretty blonde sitting at the bar with her girlfriend. I mustered up the nerve to sit close to her, and broke the ice by commenting on how unusual it was to see such a big crowd so early in the evening. She said that most of them were there for the same reason she was, and that was to take the beginner's Texas two-step class that was about to start. I saw an opportunity to get to know this woman, so I said, "Do you have a partner for the class?" When she said that she didn't, I followed with, "Would you like one?" She said, "Yes, I would."

It didn't take me long to figure out that Joann was interested in me, because she held my hand while we stood listening to the instructor. Asking her out after the lesson was easy, because I felt sure that she was going to say yes—which she did.

If you take private lessons from a studio, keep your dance instructor under control. Some studios train men and women for exhibition dancing, and they might tell you that you have great potential and suggest that you get in a training program to prepare for an exhibition. That might sound like fun, but there are some potential problems with this type of training. If the dance you specialize in is difficult for a woman to do unless she has had lessons, it will not be a useful tool for meeting women. In addition, it would probably be more useful for you to be competent in a variety of dances before you become an expert in any one.

In order to avoid getting sidetracked with specialized training, tell the instructor that the reason you are taking lessons is to be able to meet women and that you want to learn only the dances that are easy for the woman to follow. Also tell your instructor that you want to develop a good lead so the woman will look and feel good on the dance floor. Make it clear that you don't want to learn any dances where the woman has to have had lessons in that dance to be able to do it. For example, West Coast Swing is a beautiful dance, but the woman's part is complex, and many of the woman's styling moves that make the dance so beautiful to watch are done without guidance from the man. Most women in singles dance places will not have had West Coast Swing lessons, and without these lessons, a woman won't be able to follow you, no matter how good your lead.

WHERE CAN I TAKE LESSONS?

Sometimes inexpensive dance lessons are provided by:

♦ The YMCA
♦ City parks and recreation departments

♦ Adult enrichment schools
♦ Singles bars (before the regular dancing begins for the evening)

If you decide to learn from a studio, look in the yellow pages under "Dance Instruction." You might find two categories: "Ballet, Tap, Jazz, Etc." and "Ballroom and Social." You want "Ballroom and Social." Most studios provide both group and private lessons. You might also find an instructor listed who is working out of his or her home. Such an instructor will have a lower overhead, and therefore might charge less than a studio.

Talk to several studios and instructors. Find out what they teach and compare their prices. Some studios will insist that you sign a contract and will promise to make you the all-time champion of dance. That may sound great, but compare prices before deciding. Other studios won't require a contract; instead, they will teach you one level of one dance for one price. Here is what the brochure from such a studio might look like:

Rachel's Dance Studio
Schedule of Classes
Classes Continue for 5 Consecutive Weeks
No Partner Necessary

Starting Date	Dance	Instructor	Class Level	Time	Cost for 5 Weeks
Monday, Feb 12	Latin Technique	Rachel	9	7:15–8:15	$42
	Country-Western	Dan	3	7:15–8:15	$37
	Fox-Trot	Rachel	2	8:15–9:15	$37
Tuesday, Feb 13	West Coast Swing	Dan	5	7:15–8:30	$42
	Cha-Cha	Dan	5	8:45–9:45	$42
	West Coast Swing	Julia	2	7:15–8:30	$37
	Jitterbug	Julia	1	8:30–9:30	$37

Wednesday, Feb 14	Cha-Cha General	Marty	1	7:15–8:15	$37
	Ballroom Nightclub	Marty	1	8:30–9:30	$37
	Two-Step	Dan	4	7:15–8:15	$42
Thursday, Feb 15	Country-Western	Julia	1	7:15–8:30	$37
	Rumba	Marty	7	7:15–8:15	$42
	Waltz	Marty	7	8:15–9:15	$42
Friday, Feb 16	West Coast Swing	Dan	1	7:15–8:30	$37
	Foxy Slow	Marty	1	7:30–8:30	$42

You can see from this brochure for Rachel's Dance Studio that there are various levels of dance lessons. The level 1 classes are for beginners. You can continue taking lessons to very advanced levels. For example, in the brochure there is a level 9 class in Latin technique, a level 7 class in waltz, and a level 7 class in rumba. If the place you are going to meet women plays a variety of music that calls for a variety of different dances, it would probably be wise for you to go no further than level 2 in any particular dance, and then take the level 1 lessons in another dance. What you want to do is to be able to ask a woman to dance, no matter what music is being played, and then stay on the dance floor with her if a change in the music calls for another style of dance. By the time you have completed level 2 of a dance, you should be comfortable with the basic rhythm and footwork, and you will be able to lead at least a half-dozen different turns.

WILL I HAVE TO PRACTICE, OR WILL THE LESSONS ALONE BE ENOUGH?

Practice is an absolutely vital part of learning to dance. If you go for your second lesson without having practiced what you learned in the first, you will be struggling, and you won't enjoy it. It is much more effective to go dancing between lessons and practice what you have learned. Then you will be ready for the new material in the next lesson.

Because you and all the women in the class are going to need to practice, you will have the perfect opportunity to get to know any woman in the class you choose. Pick out the one you would most like to meet and say, "I'll never learn this unless I practice. Would you be interested in going to a dance spot to practice with me some night this week?" That's an easy date to make. If none of the women in the class interest you romantically, ask one of them anyway. Practice will make you both better dancers.

You may think that you can't learn to dance because you don't have a sense of rhythm; many men feel that way. You probably have a good sense of rhythm, but you might need some practice to bring it out. A great way to work on your sense of rhythm is to practice dancing alone in the privacy of your home. That is what Troy did, and it helped him a lot:

> I have joint custody of my daughter. I love it because Katie spends a lot of time at my house, but when I have her with me, I can't get out to the singles spots where I might meet a woman. I decided to put this "home time" to good use by practicing what I am learning in my dance lessons. Now when Katie is outside playing with her friends, I put the music on good and loud, hold my arms up in dance position as if I were leading a woman, and then I dance, practicing the steps and leading the turns.
>
> When I first tried practicing alone, I felt silly. Katie made a few wisecracks about it too, which didn't help. But now it is just part of my daily routine. It is relaxing and good exercise, and it has definitely improved my dancing. Practicing at home is helping me develop a sense of rhythm, and moves that feel smooth and natural.

When you start feeling the rhythm and getting the moves down, the dancing bug may bite you. Many people who start out just trying to learn a simple dance get completely swept away by it. These people sometimes wind up making dance the center of their lives. It all starts with the first dance lesson, and practice.

Paul, a friend of ours, discovered that the better he got at dancing, the more confident he became about asking women to dance, so he took more lessons and practiced, and eventually became a highly skilled dancer. Here is what Paul told us about how being a good dancer helped him meet Angela, the woman he is with today:

I met Angela at a singles dance. While we were dancing, she told me she lived in Fort Collins. I thought to myself, "I don't do Fort Collins; that's a ninety-minute drive." I couldn't see myself getting involved with a woman who lived so far away, but she was cute and a wonderful dancer, so when I left her, I gave her my card and said, "If you would like to go dancing sometime, give me a call." A week later she called and said, "There's a big dance coming up in Fort Collins in two weeks. Would you like to go?" It sounded like fun, so I drove up to Fort Collins for the dance. I had such a great time with her that I decided I did do Fort Collins. We dated for a year, and then she lost her job and moved in with me.

Here is what Angela said about how she met Paul:

The night I met Paul I wasn't out trying to meet a man. I had just broken up with a man, and the last thing I wanted to do was jump back into a relationship. I was just out that night to have fun dancing. I danced with several men that night. Paul was by far the best dancer.

When Paul left, he gave me his card and asked me to call him if I ever wanted to go dancing. A few days later I learned about a dance that was coming up that would have a live band playing forties music. Paul seemed to be able to dance to just about any music, so I thought he would be a good partner for the forties dance. When I called him and asked him if he would like to go, he seemed really hesitant. But he finally agreed, and we had a great time at the dance. We danced to every song played.

Just as the longest journey begins with the first step, becoming a good dancer begins with the first lesson. If you do nothing else recommended in this book, at least do one thing: Sign up for dance lessons. It is an excellent way to meet women and get dates, and taking a woman out to dance on the first date makes for a very romantic evening. The money you spend on dance lessons could easily be the best investment you ever make.

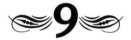

Five Mistakes to Avoid

One of the keys to getting better at meeting women is to recognize if and when you are making a mistake. If you don't realize that you are doing something wrong, you will probably keep repeating that error. Here are five mistakes commonly made by men when they are trying to meet women. Analyze your behavior to see if you are making any of these mistakes, and if so, try to change your behavior.

MISTAKE NO. 1—WAITING TO GET YOUR NERVE UP

When a typical man sees a woman he would like to meet, he usually doesn't immediately approach her. Instead he hangs back, waiting to get his nerve up. There are three problems with doing this: It doesn't work, it wastes your time, and you might lose your chance to meet her.

Wouldn't it be great if waiting to get your nerve up did work? Then, no matter how gorgeous the woman, all you would have to do is stay put for a while, getting braver and braver, until eventually you could boldly approach her. But usually after a man spends a long time in agony waiting to get his nerve up, he is no braver than he was before. Actually, he might be even less likely to approach the woman, because as he sits there gazing at her and fantasizing about her, he begins to fall in love. When that happens, he no longer faces being rejected by a stranger, he now faces being rejected by someone he is starting to have feelings for, and that makes the approach more difficult. The waiting accomplishes nothing.

Besides being ineffective, waiting to get your nerve up has a couple of undesirable side effects. While you are delaying your approach, the woman may leave, or she may be approached by another man who then monopolizes her time. In addition, it is a waste of time to agonize a long time over approaching a woman. She might not even want to meet you. The sooner you find out that she is *not* interested in you, the sooner you can spend your time looking for a woman who *is* interested.

Harvey, one of our students, realized that he always made the mistake of waiting to get his nerve up, and he decided to change his behavior. This is what he told us:

> You told me what a waste of time it was to wait a long time to get my nerve up before approaching a woman. I realized this was something I always did, so I adopted a new strategy. Now when I see a woman I want to meet, I won't allow myself even one minute of worry time. Instead, I say to myself, "Feet, don't fail me now," and I immediately start walking in her direction. I usually don't have the rest of my plan in place yet, I just start moving. It's amazing how effective it is. I get on my feet and get closer to the woman so I can say something if the opportunity arises.

Because waiting is counterproductive, when you see a woman you would like to meet, immediately find a way to get near her so you can be in a position to start a conversation. It might not be easy, but the more you do it the easier it will become.

Mistake No. 2—Failing to Ask for a Date at the First Opportunity

This is another time-wasting behavior that has a downside. Here is what happened to Jonathan when he put off asking Rose for a date:

I know that you can meet women in adult enrichment classes, so I signed up for "Healthy East Indian Cooking," a Monday-night class that would run for three weeks.

As I headed down the hall to the first class, I overtook a young lady who was also taking the class. I introduced myself and struck up a brief conversation. I knew almost immediately that I wanted to ask Rose out. I managed to talk to her several more times during the class, and at the end of the class, I walked her to her car. She sat on the hood of her car, and we talked for a long time. I wanted desperately to ask her for a date, but I was afraid. Since I was going to see her in two more classes, I decided that I could wait and ask her out later. Since we would know each other better by then, it would be easier to ask for a date. So I didn't ask her out. I just said good night.

At the next class I watched the door anxiously, waiting for Rose to show up, but she never did. I was disappointed, but I realized that she might have missed the class because she was sick. I thought I might still have a chance to ask her out when she came to the final class, but she didn't show up for that class either.

I wondered if she might have dropped the class because there was nobody there who interested her, including me. Then I had an even worse thought. I wondered if I might have been the only guy in the class who interested her, and she didn't come back because after we had talked for so long and I didn't ask her out, she thought that I wasn't interested in her.

By failing to ask Rose out after the first class, Jonathan made a mistake, and it cost him a chance to date a woman he liked. Don't make the same mistake Jonathan did. Ask a woman for a date the first time you are with her. Returning to a place again and again, hoping to see her, creates a lot of unnecessary anxiety and is not an effective use of your time.

MISTAKE NO. 3—FAILING TO GET HER NUMBER

After talking with a woman for some period of time, you will need to decide whether you want to ask her out. Sometimes the answer is definitely yes, sometimes definitely no, and sometimes you are undecided. When you are undecided, we recommend that you always get her number. Ken told us a story that shows why:

Last year I spent four months in Guam on business. Sitting next to me on the flight to Guam was a young woman who was a native of Guam. She had been working in the United States for two years and was returning to Guam to live. She was nice enough, but I didn't get her number because I've never had a problem meeting women, and I figured I would meet a lot of women when I got to Guam. However, soon after I arrived, I learned that there were seventy-thousand military personnel on Guam (mostly men) and a population of only thirty-thousand natives. Women of any kind were in high demand. When you would approach a woman in a grocery store at 10:00 A.M., she would act as if it was the third time she had been approached that day (and it might have been). I went four months without a date. I often wondered what my stay would have been like if I had asked the young lady on the plane for a number where I could reach her.

When you have an opportunity to get a woman's number, get it. Once you have her number, you can choose to call her or not. When you don't have her number, you are out of luck. You can't call her even if you want to.

Mistake No. 4—Making Assumptions

When a man sees a woman he would like to meet, he usually makes a judgment about the odds that she will go out with him. In many cases a man will say to himself, "She's too beautiful—she wouldn't want to go out with me." He then decides against trying to meet her.

When a man assumes that a woman wouldn't want to meet him, he has found an excuse for not facing potential rejection. Since the outcome of the venture is already known, there is no sense in experiencing the pain of failure, right?

Be aware of how assumptions of this nature can prevent you from meeting the women you desire the most. When you assume that a woman doesn't want to meet you, you will guess wrong some of the time. Assumptions of this nature are the worst example of shooting yourself in the foot. The rule we follow is: **Don't make assumptions. Get the facts.**

The way to get the facts is to approach a woman, talk to her, and ask her out. There is something very satisfying about getting the doubts out of your mind by getting the facts. If you don't talk to a woman and ask her out, you will never know what her answer would have been. Although it may be difficult for you to approach a woman and ask for a date, you will be rewarded when you do, no matter what her answer is. Even when a woman turns you down, you will be proud of yourself for trying. After you have been turned down, POOF, she will disappear from your thoughts and you can then concentrate on meeting someone else.

Mistake No. 5—Reading Body Language

Many books for single men have entire chapters on how to read a woman's body language. These books have long lists of both positive and negative body language, and some suggest that you not approach a woman unless she sends you a positive signal. Positive signals listed in one book were licking lips (her own), stroking her hair or face, a head toss, a smile, a glance at you that lingers before she looks away, and legs crossed with knees pointed in your direction. Negative body language included folded arms, clenched fists, an expressionless face, and standing with ankles crossed.

Ignore this advice. We have found that reading body language is worse than useless, it is counterproductive. When you attempt to interpret a woman's body language, you have to make assumptions, and to avoid rejection, you may assume that the body language from an attractive women is negative.

A woman may be happy, sad, lonely, warm, or cold. Her body language will probably reflect how she is feeling more than how she feels about *you*. Most women will not be trying to send you a message. Even if women did send out clear signals, they would be basing their decision only on your looks. After you start talking to a woman, you let her see a bit of your personality. Often it's a man's personality that convinces a woman to go out with him. For example, we were at a dance one evening, sharing a table with a group of women, when one of them saw a man looking at her and said, "Oh God! I think that guy is going to ask me to dance. I don't want to meet him." Well, the guy did ask her to dance, and she accepted just to be nice. After several dances she returned to our table and said, "You know, I really *like* that guy." Later in the evening she accepted a date with him. If that man had waited for a nonverbal clue before asking her to dance, they wouldn't have met.

If you are trying to meet a woman in a nonsingles place such as a grocery store or post office, she may not even be aware of your presence. How will she send you any kind of signal when she doesn't even know that you are there? Ignore body language. The only way to know if a woman is interested in you is to talk to her.

When you don't approach a woman because you think that her body language is negative, you are just caving in to the fear of rejection. What you should be doing is training yourself to overcome this fear. Don't try to read a woman's body language, just complete the Five Steps.

Now that you are aware of these common mistakes, try to avoid them. The more you avoid them, the more success you will have meeting women and getting dates.

≈ **10** ≈

Training Aids

When we ask the men in our class (and other men) what their biggest problem is in meeting women, they almost always say, "The fear of rejection," or "The fear of approaching women." We wish we had a pill men could take that would eliminate this fear. We could sell the pills worldwide. We would be millionaires, and the world would be full of Don Juans. Unfortunately, there is no such pill, so if you have a strong fear of rejection that prevents you from meeting women, you will have to overcome the fear on your own. You may not believe it now, but with training, you can do it. The results will be the same as with our pill—it will just take longer.

You don't have to train until the fear is entirely gone, only until it is reduced to a level where you can meet women in spite of the fear. Gradually, after a period of training, when you see an attractive woman you want to meet, instead of feeling an immobilizing fear, you will feel a little fear mixed with a little tingle of excitement. It will be like what our friend Joe, an army paratrooper, now feels when he jumps out of airplanes:

> On my first jump I was scared to death. I stood in the doorway of the plane and was so scared I didn't hear the jump master screaming at me to go. He finally had to kick me in the pants to get me out the door. After that, it got easier on each

jump. But I don't want the fear to go away completely, because now I find the fear exciting.

Think about it this way; you might have a huge fear of rejection, but you probably also have a tremendous desire to have a woman in your life. Right now, your fear might be too big for your desire to overcome. On a bar chart it might look like this, with the bar for fear slightly taller.

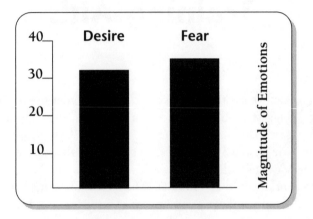

After a period of self-training, the bar chart might look like this:

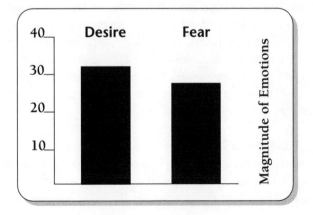

Your desire is the same as before, but with the fear slightly reduced, your desire is now dominant. If you have a strong desire to have a woman in your life, a small reduction in fear might be all it takes to allow you to meet the women you want to meet. You don't have to completely eliminate your fear, you just have to reduce it. To help you reduce your fear we have developed the following training aids.

Aid No. 1—Contrary Training

Inside us all there is a little voice of fear. It means well; it is there to protect us. It keeps us from going into the jungle at night when the big cats are hunting, and it keeps us from standing near the edge of a cliff from which we could fall. But when it comes to meeting women, the little voice of fear really gets in the way. It is hard to understand why it is so strong. Perhaps it had some survival value in primitive times when approaching a desirable woman might have led to a fight with her mate, but nobody really knows. It is a rare man indeed, however, who does not hear this little voice of fear when he faces approaching an attractive woman.

When you are out somewhere trying to meet a woman, you will often hear the little voice, and not just when you see a desirable woman. For example, you might be in a dance spot early in the evening when there is a crowd, but the dance floor is empty and you want to go to the other side of the room. The shortest route would be to walk across the empty dance floor, but the little voice will say, "Don't do that—people are watching—you will be conspicuous out there all alone." Then you will take the longer route through the crowd. This situation is perfect for contrary training. As soon as you hear the little voice of fear telling you to do one thing, do the exact opposite; that is what contrary training is. As soon as you hear the little voice telling you not to cross the dance floor with people watching, walk right across the dance floor.

Stuart, one of our students, found a chance to use contrary training at work. Here is what he told us:

One day when I walked into the auditorium for a presentation, I saw a really great-looking woman I had seen in the halls, but had never met. I had heard that she was married, but I wanted to find out for sure. She was sitting in the front row, alone. In the back row there were several men. I could sit anywhere I wanted, and I wanted to sit next to the attractive woman, but I heard the little voice of fear telling me to play it safe and sit with the men. The little voice told me the woman would think it was kind of strange if I took the seat right next to her. The little voice also told me that if I walked up front and sat next to the woman, the men in the back of the room would be watching me. But then I remembered what you are supposed to do when you hear that little voice of fear telling you to play it safe. I realized that this was a perfect opportunity for some contrary training, so I walked right up front and sat beside her. At first I felt awkward, and I sensed that I had made her feel uneasy too, but I quickly introduced myself, and pretty soon she was smiling and talking. It turned out she was married. But I was proud of myself for sitting next to her and showing the voice of fear who was boss.

Each time that you use contrary training you will be making only a small change in your behavior, but over time these small changes add up.

AID NO. 2—CHALLENGE TRAINING

Not all of the situations where you want to approach a woman and get a date will be of the same difficulty. Some approaches will be harder because of the woman's beauty, where she is standing, or whom she is with. Instead of passing up an opportunity to meet a woman because you are uneasy about the approach, realize that you are in training, and think of a difficult approach as an opportunity to improve. Once you force yourself to meet a woman under challenging conditions, a normal approach will seem easy.

Here is a story from a former student of ours who accepted an exceptionally tough challenge as part of his training program:

I was in a singles bar early one evening when seven good-looking young ladies came in together and took seats on bar stools facing the empty dance floor. I would have been happy to meet any one of them, but with the dance floor empty, I knew it was a long shot whether any of them would want to dance. Then I realized that I was faced with a challenging situation, and to improve, I had to accept such challenges, so I asked the young lady at one end of the group if she would like to dance. She said, "No, thank you." I then took a step to the side, and asked her friend. Again, "No, thank you." I felt that the rest of the women were not likely to accept the first two women's leftovers, but I was on a training mission, so I continued down the line until I had been rejected by all seven, with everyone in the place watching. Then an interesting thing happened. A woman on an upper level must have felt sorry for me, because she called out, "I'll dance with you." The two of us got the action started on the dance floor.

After that experience, asking a woman to dance became just a little bit easier than it was before. Why should I be afraid of a single rejection when I knew I could handle seven?

Aid No. 3—Cross Training

One of the questions asked most frequently by the men in our class is, "What do you say to meet a woman in a supermarket?" When a man asks that question, we don't tell him what to say. We know that if we told him what to say, he probably still wouldn't approach a woman in the supermarket, because his real problem is not that he doesn't know what to say, his real problem is that he is afraid. So when a man asks that question, we surprise him with our answer. We say, "If you want to be able to meet a woman in the supermarket, go to the singles dance bars," and then we give him the following explanation of our concept of cross training.

When your problem is a lack of nerve, you simply need more practice meeting women, and the best place to practice is somewhere where there are a lot of easy meeting opportunities. Despite the fact that many men say they hate singles bars and singles events, these are excellent places to practice meeting women. For example, in a singles bar with dancing, all you have to do is say, "Would you like to dance?" and you will have a woman in your arms ready, and actually expecting, to talk with you. At a singles mixer you will find women either standing alone or in small conversation groups, hoping some man will come over and start a conversation. Although you might find starting a conversation at a mixer more difficult than asking a woman to dance, once you get up the nerve to do it, there will be endless opportunities to practice.

Once you have progressed to the point where you can easily meet woman at singles bars or singles mixers, you will be much better prepared to start a conversation with a woman in other places, such as a supermarket. That is the concept of cross training. You train in a place where it is easy to meet women, then you apply your new-found skills in another, more difficult place.

We have a friend, Barry, who told us how the practice he got in the singles places helped him develop the skill to meet women anywhere.

There was a time when I couldn't meet women at all, and I went for years without a girlfriend. How I hated those years. Eventually I started going to singles bars. At first I wasn't very good at meeting women there, but I went a lot, and over time, I got better at it. Then I started going to singles mixers a couple of times a week. At first, I was pretty hopeless. I just couldn't bring myself to approach an attractive woman in that environment and start a conversation, but again I went a lot, and after a while I developed enough nerve to be able to meet women there too. The skill I developed in singles bars and singles mixers has really helped me, because now when I look back on where I met the women I have dated recently, it turns out I have met them in all sorts of different places. I dated a salesgirl I met in a store, I dated a woman I met at the beach, I dated a woman I met in a restaurant, and I dated a woman I met while riding my bike in a park. I guess I can meet women just about anywhere now. Let me tell you, the ability to meet women is a skill worth developing. Being alone is no fun.

Although Barry didn't call it cross training, that is exactly what he was doing as he developed his skill at meeting women. He started out in singles bars, and after he was comfortable there, he branched out to singles mixers. The training he got meeting women in those singles places prepared him for meeting women in nonsingles places such as stores and restaurants. Today Barry can meet women anywhere he goes. He wasn't born with that ability—he trained himself to have it.

AID NO. 4—THE GRADING SYSTEM

One of the problems with training yourself to meet women is you have to be your own coach. Nobody else will be pressuring you to practice, and nobody else will be judging your progress—you have to do it all. And because there is no final exam coming up, it will be tempting to just keep doing things the way you always have. If your problem is that you are afraid to approach an attractive woman and start a conversation, it will be easy to just keep hanging back, wishing you had the nerve to make an approach. If you can talk to women, but you find it very difficult to ask for a date, it will be easy to keep failing in that area too.

We have a grading system that might help you get better at meeting women. This is how our grading system works: After you have been out somewhere trying to meet women and are on your way home, grade yourself on that outing. At first you might think, "Well, last time I was out looking I failed to get a date, so I must get an F." That's not what the grading system is about at all. With our grading system, you grade your behavior, not the results.

For example, if during the course of an evening, you found three women you wanted to meet, eventually got into conversations with each one, asked each one out, and got three rejections, you would get an A. You did everything you could—you completed the Five Steps with every woman you wanted to meet. If, on the other hand, you met the three women and talked with each one for a while, but didn't ask any of them out because you were afraid, you would get maybe a C. You don't get an F because you were out there trying, but you certainly can't give yourself an A when you chickened out on the close.

The grading system does not have to be fixed; it can change with time. If the first time you go out you fail to talk to any of the women you want to meet, a C might be okay because at least you are out there with the intention of meeting women. Maybe you are new at it and are having a tough time. But if you have gone out ten times and are still not approaching the women you would like to meet, it is time to get harder on yourself. The C should go to a D for a few outings, and then finally to an F. What you are telling yourself is, "Don't keep hanging back! Don't keep making that same mistake, stupid!"

With our grading system you give yourself the grade, but there is still a way you can use this system with a friend. If you have a friend who is also trying to meet women, you can ask one another, "What kind of grade did you get the last time you were out looking?" If, while you are out looking, you know that you are going to have to face your friend and tell him your grade on that outing, it might give you the little boost you need to change your behavior and avoid confessing to a low grade.

Eugene learned about our grading system when he took our class. He later told us that the system did make him improve, and faster than he ever expected. Here is what happened to him:

I had been going to a singles club dance every Friday for a long time, and I was getting better at asking women to dance, but I still couldn't bring myself to ask a woman for a date. I thought that I would probably get turned down, and that would hurt, so I didn't ask. Then one Friday night I danced with a woman whom I really wanted to get to know. After a few songs, I escorted her back to her seat and left her alone, just as I always did when I was through dancing. I wanted to ask her for a date, but I was afraid. Then I had a brilliant idea: I would ask her to meet me at the dance the next Friday. Since she was probably going to be there anyway, she wasn't likely to say no. If she would meet me there the next Friday, we could dance some more and get to know one another better. Maybe then it would be easier to ask her for a date.

With this plan in mind I went over and again asked her to dance. Again she accepted, and again we chatted while we danced. After a few numbers, I walked her back to her table, and as I was getting ready to leave, I put my plan into action by saying, "Do you come here often?" But she replied, "Practically never." How was I supposed to say I would meet her there again the next week when she says something like that? So I just thanked her for the dance and left.

As I was driving home I remembered the grading system and reviewed my performance to see what grade I should get. I thought to myself, "When I asked her to dance, she danced with me. While we danced she smiled and laughed at my jokes. When I asked her to dance a second time she danced with me. Now I am driving home alone and she is still back there trying to meet a man. You get an F, you coward. You do this every time."

I was really upset with my lousy performance, and the more I thought about it, the madder I got. Then, all of a sudden, I made a U-turn and headed back to the dance. When I went in, she was still there. Again I asked her to dance, and again she accepted, but this time when we were through dancing, I was a changed man—I just wasn't going to screw this up again. Instead of taking her back to her table and leaving, I asked her if she would like to meet me for lunch the next day. She agreed and gave me her number.

The grading system helps you to be your own coach. It forces you to analyze your performance after each outing, and it helps you keep pressure on yourself to improve. If you are going out looking, but you keep making the same mistakes, do what Eugene did in the above story: Get angry at yourself, and give yourself a big fat F. After that, get very determined that you are going to start getting better grades.

The grading system can also help you get over the disappointment you feel when a woman rejects your offer of a date. You may not have gotten a date, but if you did all the necessary steps, getting an A might help you feel better.

Getting better at meeting women and getting dates is a gradual process that takes some time. These four training aids might speed up your rate of improvement. We recommend that you use them all as often as you can.

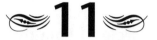

The Rule of One Hundred

When we ask the men in our class how often they go out trying to meet women, a few will say they go out once or twice a week, but most say they never go out with the specific intent of meeting a woman. One man said, "I go bowling once a week, does that count?"

Another said, "I stay home so much I have practically become a hermit." Craig, told the class how he spends his spare time:

> I spent last weekend loading ammo and playing with my dog. My last date was a year ago—a friend fixed me up. I'm waiting for my friends to fix me up again. I never go out trying to meet women anymore. I tried it a few times and it was hard on my ego; it seems the women are just out there to reject men. Now I let my friends pre-filter the women for me.

There are many good single men who, like Craig, seldom go out trying to meet women because they hate what they have to go through. But because they don't try, their skill at meeting women doesn't improve. Because they aren't good at meeting women and because they seldom try, they don't get dates. These men are trapped in what we call the Circle of Failure.

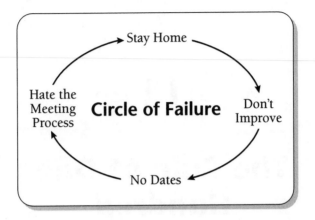

Even though Craig dislikes going out to meet women, actually going out and trying is the only way to break out of the Circle of Failure. When he didn't have any success, Craig *decreased* his effort. Instead, he should have *increased* his effort. By trying harder, over time Craig would get better at meeting women, and he would begin to get dates. Then he would begin to tolerate the process of meeting women. That would make him willing to go out more often, and when he did, he would get even better at meeting women. Craig's Circle of Failure would then have turned into his Circle of Success.

We have a friend, Clint, who has moved from the Circle of Fail-

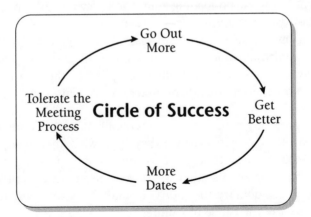

ure to the Circle of Success. When we saw Clint about a year ago, we asked him how his love life was. He replied:

> Not too good, actually. I'm pretty lonely, but being lonely is better than the rejection I was experiencing when I was trying to meet girls. Now I just stay home. I have my books; I have my TV. I don't need the rejection.

Clint seemed bitter about his lack of success with women and all the rejection he had experienced. We talked Clint into taking our course on how to get a date. After hearing the other men in the class tell about their experiences, Clint saw that he wasn't the only man who had experienced a lot of rejection. Clint decided to give it another try. He took dance lessons and went to singles dances spots a lot. When we checked back with him a few months later, he had a different story to tell:

> I've learned a lot in the last few months. It was really tough in the beginning. I had a terrible time getting up the nerve to ask a woman to dance, and when I got turned down, it really hurt. But despite the pain, I just kept going out, night after night. After a while, I learned that even though I get turned down a lot, I occasionally get accepted, and that has made it easier. A few months ago I wouldn't have believed this would ever happen, but I'm starting to enjoy all the socializing in the dance spots, and I am meeting women and going out on dates.

Even though Clint has been going out for several months now and is starting to get dates, he is still not in an intimate relationship. That is not an unusual situation; it often takes a while to find a woman who is a really good match for you.

We know a man, Lance, who moved into the Circle of Success. Even though Lance is good at meeting women, there are still periods when he doesn't have a girlfriend. Lance told us that he has a theory on how often he has to go out to find a woman who will be right for a long-term relationship:

It has been my experience that on any one outing to a place or event, I have only a very small chance that I will meet a woman who will be right for a long-term relationship. I figure that my chance of meeting this woman on any one outing is something like one in a hundred. Therefore, I estimate that I might have to make one hundred outings before I find her.

Since I don't like being without a woman, I try to go to one hundred places in as short a time as possible. I have discovered that by giving it the maximum effort, I can go to one hundred places in about a month. This system works for me. I seldom go more than a month without a woman in my life.

We agree with Lance's philosophy. A man can expect to make a lot of outings before he is likely to meet a woman with whom everything works. In our class, we have adopted Lance's philosophy, and we tell the men that if they want to get into a relationship, they should be prepared to make about one hundred outings. We call this the Rule of One Hundred.

Of course, there is nothing magic about the number one hundred. We use it in our class because it is a big number that makes the impression that meeting the right woman can require a major effort. The Rule of One Hundred is meant to be a motivator, not a law of science.

Lance provided us with his activities calendar for one week to show us what a typical week of his maximum-effort schedule is like:

Sunday (7 Outings)
Church.
Church singles brunch.
Bike ride in park.
Stroll through mall, snack at mall food court.
Adult enrichment class group tour of historic homes.
Dinner at popular singles restaurant with outdoor deck.
Singles discussion group.

Monday (4 outings)
Health club before work.
Lunch at salad bar.
Adult enrichment class on meeting other singles (over at 8:30 P.M.).
A singles bar with dancing.

Tuesday (4 outings)
Eat sandwich in park, walk around lake.
Dinner at a downtown "sit and read" coffeehouse that has sidewalk tables.
Ballroom dance lessons.
A singles bar with dancing.

Wednesday (4 outings)
Health club before work.
Lunch at cafeteria near hospital (where the doctors and nurses eat).
Singles mixer (with buffet) after work.
A singles bar with dancing.

Thursday (4 outings)
Walk mall at noon, eat at mall food court.
Dinner at a cafeteria.
Western dance lessons.
A singles bar with dancing.

Friday (5 outings)
Health club before work.
Lunch at fast food outlet near office buildings.
Happy hour and dinner at a popular microbrewery.
Singles club dance.
Two singles bars.

Saturday (6 outings)
Breakfast in coffeehouse.
Health club.
Lunch in park and walk around lake.
Bike ride (on path by large condo developments).
Pizza (at the pizza parlor near the teachers' college).
Three singles bars with dancing.

You will notice that this maximum-effort schedule doesn't allow much time for you to hang out with your friends or to stay home and watch TV. If you follow a schedule such as this, it will force you to live your life outside of your house, out there where single women are.

You might have also noticed that Lance has a lot of singles bars on his schedule. He said that when he has nothing else scheduled, he uses singles bars as schedule "fillers." Note also that the restaurants on Lance's schedule are places where you seat yourself, such as salad bars, cafeterias, and coffeehouses. He prefers these because he can take a seat near any woman he wants to meet.

Lance was able to maintain this schedule with a full-time professional career. However, this maximum effort program assumes that you don't have additional time-consuming obligations such as parenting or getting a degree. Such obligations may reduce the time you have to meet women, but not necessarily eliminate it. Much of Lance's effort took advantage of time spent in everyday activities such as eating meals and working out. Possibly you could combine meeting someone with your daily activities. If you are a single parent, the possibility of meeting a woman on an outing with your children exists. Many places you would take your children offer opportunities to meet single mothers. If you are getting a degree, consider trying to meet women in class, on campus, or while studying in the library. A "maximum effort" may not be feasible for you, but, with some thought, you can probably increase your present effort and your chances of success.

With a schedule like that you also need enough money to eat out, take dance lessons, and take adult enrichment classes. If such a cost is too much for you, use some imagination and substitute other outings that are less expensive or free.

If you have never been on such a maximum-effort program, you might think that it is not realistic, but it is. It will take a total commitment on your part to get on such a schedule and stay on it, but you can do it. Other men have. This program really works, and it has some side benefits as well:

♦ If you are just coming out of a relationship, you probably feel sad and lonely. A crash schedule will keep you so busy you won't have time to mope around feeling sorry for yourself.

♦ When you are at one event trying to meet a woman, and you have two other places that you want to hit before you go home, you are under time pressure. Sometimes this pressure makes you get up and approach a woman instead of hanging back.

♦ A maximum-effort schedule will help reduce your fear of rejection. If you are going out only once a week trying to meet a woman, you have an awful lot riding on the outcome of any one approach. With a maximum-effort schedule, each meeting opportunity is less critical, and you can be more relaxed and confident when you approach a woman. You can say to yourself, "If this doesn't work out, I will get another chance at the next place."

♦ A maximum-effort schedule is the best way to get better fast. When you do something wrong in one place, you will remember your mistake when going on to the next place, and therefore you will be less likely to repeat it. With such a schedule, you won't get rusty between outings.

Because following the Rule of One Hundred maximum-effort program is complicated, we recommend that you keep an activities calendar. An activities calendar will help with both long-range and short-range planning.

Long-Range Planning

Gather all the information you can about what is going on around town. If there are adult enrichment classes available, get the catalog of classes. If there are entertainment weeklies or singles newspapers, read them. Read the entertainment section of your daily paper. Talk to friends. Find out what events are coming up where you could go to meet women. Special events for singles are good, but you can also meet single women at events for the general public.

Now choose the events and classes you want to attend and write them on your calendar. Include lectures, adult enrichment classes, dance lessons, singles mixers, singles club meetings, and anything else that has a fixed time and date. This is your long-range plan.

SHORT-RANGE PLANNING

At the beginning of each week see where the gaps are on your calendar and fill them in with activities that you can do at any time. For example, if you see an opening on Saturday or Sunday, plan to spend part of the day at the park, mall, food court, library, or bookstore. Whatever you decide, write it on your calendar. If you see you have some evenings open, plan to go to a shopping mall, a library, or a singles bar with dancing. If you have time for an entire evening of bar hopping, decide which ones you are going to hit and in what order. Some may be better early in the evening, some later. You want to be at each singles bar at the best time, while minimizing your driving time. It may take some thought. This is your short-range planning.

Of course, you don't have to enter your short-range activities at the beginning of each week. You could plan each evening after you get home from work, but when you leave it to the last minute, it is too easy to come home, flop on the couch, flip on the TV, and veg out for the evening. When you already have the evening planned, you will be thinking about it during the day, and therefore you will be more likely to keep to your schedule.

Your chances of getting a date are directly proportional to the effort you put into it. If you go out two times a week you have twice the probability of meeting a woman compared to going out once a week. If you go out ten times a week you have ten times the probability of meeting a woman compared to going out once a week. If having a woman in your life is a top priority for you, make the maximum effort possible. This means filling up all the blank spaces on your calendar with activities for finding a mate. Any day or evening that you are home alone, there is a place or event in your city where there are available single women. You should be there.

Many lonely people feel that meeting someone to love is a matter of luck. We overheard a man tell his friend that he had been going out to a singles dance every week trying to meet a woman. His friend replied, "You're trying too hard. Just let it happen." What terrible advice. Waiting for it to "just happen" is like waiting to win the lottery without buying any tickets. Before you can win, you have to play the game.

If you are going to play the game, why stretch it out over a long time? Get it over with by filling out an activities calendar and getting busy. See if you can match Lance's feat of going to one hundred places in one month. That is a challenge that will get you going. Before the month is up you will probably see that you are getting better at meeting women, you're enjoying it more, and you might even have a new problem: so many women—so little time.

Part II

Putting Your Plan
Into Action

$\mathcal{W}$e described the Five Steps to our friend Neil and told him that if he got out and started using them, he would get better at meeting women. Neil took our advice and went to a singles mixer. This is what happened:

When I walked in, there were hundreds of people milling about. I saw a woman I wanted to meet, and I knew I was supposed to do these steps, but I didn't know how to do them at a singles mixer. I felt awkward and out of place just standing there not knowing what to do. I left after half an hour, feeling pretty bad about the whole thing.

Neil gets credit for at least getting out. If you want to meet women, getting out is essential. But Neil has a common problem. He didn't know what to do in a specific meeting situation—he didn't know how to customize the Five Steps for a particular place. If you have this problem, the next six chapters can be of help. These chapters provide the details on how experts (men experienced at meeting women in a specific situation) apply the Five Steps in that situation. The next six chapters address how to meet women:

♦ At a singles mixer
♦ While biking
♦ At a singles bar
♦ At the beach
♦ At airports and on airplanes
♦ While skiing

In each of these six meeting situations, the experts give specific techniques for applying the Five Steps. You can learn from their experience and avoid Neil's problem of "just standing there not knowing what to do."

These six chapters are not necessarily meant to be read sequentially; they are intended more as a reference. If you are going to be in one of these six meeting situations, read the appropriate chapter before you go. It will give you a refresher course on the Five Steps, with specific advice on how to apply them.

The advice in these chapters will also be useful for meeting a woman at other places. For instance, meeting women at a singles mixer is similar to meeting women in any social gathering where people are moving about, such as a street fair, convention, or wine tasting. The advice given for a singles bar can be applied to any function where there is dancing, such as a party, a wedding, or a church dance. The techniques for meeting women while biking, skiing, or at the beach may help you meet women at other outdoor activities. Knowing how to meet women at airports and on airplanes may help you meet women while traveling by subway, bus, train, or ship.

We are not necessarily recommending these six places as the best places for you to go. You may be more successful in other places (anyplace is a good place if there are women there and you know how to meet them). We do recommend that you read these chapters, however, and learn from the experts. You may get ideas and inspiration (applying the Five Steps sometimes takes creativity). Remember, at one time these experts were novices. Using the trial and error method, they gradually learned how to meet women. Take advantage of their experience and avoid the slow, and sometimes painful, learning process.

❧12❧

How to Meet a Woman at a Singles Mixer

*A*ny event that caters to singles and that has a cocktail-party atmosphere can be called a "singles mixer." A hotel in our city holds a singles mixer once a year that is billed as "the world's largest office party." Well over a thousand people attend this event where singles mill around with drinks in hand trying to meet the opposite sex. Such events provide abundant meeting opportunities for men who have the knowledge and skills to meet women in such an environment. The purpose of this chapter is to give you such expertise. The techniques presented can be used at other stand-up social gatherings, such as conferences, charity benefits, wine tastings, and intermissions during concerts or plays.

Advantage of Singles Mixers
At a mixer there are usually a large number of women, most of whom are single and there to meet a man. There are few other places with so many single women.

Disadvantages of Singles Mixers
Single mixers have a meat-market atmosphere. Men and women are there for one reason—to meet someone of the opposite sex. For most men it's not easy to start a conversation and get a date in such

115

a contrived atmosphere. If you don't know what to do at a mixer, you can spend hours eyeing the women, without getting one number.

When to Go—How Long to Stay

Singles mixers are usually scheduled to catch the after-work crowd. Mixers often start about four in the afternoon and end around eight. Some women drop in right after work. Others go home first and arrive at the mixer later. Because women will be coming and going all evening, there is no best time to show up. We recommend that you go early and stay late, though, because the longer you are there applying the Five Steps, the better chance you have of meeting a woman.

THE FIVE STEPS AT A SINGLES MIXER

At a mixer there is usually no one to introduce you to a woman you want to meet—you are on your own. You must approach a woman "cold turkey," start a conversation, and, after talking for a while, ask her out. Most men don't do this very well. As a result, even though you may see hundreds of single men and women at a mixer trying to meet someone, you seldom see phone numbers being exchanged. Knowing what to do at a singles mixer can make all the difference. Drawing on our own experience at singles mixers, we have customized the Five Steps for this environment.

Step 1—Search

At singles mixers you will often see groups of men standing together talking. Occasionally one of the men will look over his shoulder to see if there are any appealing women nearby. Occasionally looking over your shoulder is not an effective search strategy. A good search strategy is a focused activity that lets you choose from all (or at least most) of the women there, not just from the few who happen to be nearby.

When to Search

Actively searching can make you feel conspicuous; therefore, you might have a tendency to stand around talking to your buddies while you wait to get your nerve up. This doesn't work. Searching will not be any easier after talking to your friends for an hour than it would have been the minute you walked in the door. As a matter of fact, searching is usually more difficult after a long delay because you are then in the habit of doing nothing. When you walk in the door you are in an active mode. Stay in that mode. Get a drink if you want, but then immediately begin to search. After all, the reason you are there is to meet a woman, and the logical first step is to find her. Every minute you delay your search, you decrease your chances of meeting that special woman. She might leave or get into a conversation with another man. There is no reason to postpone the start of your search. The embarrassing feeling that "everyone will know what I am doing" will fade with experience. Besides, most people at a singles mixer are too concerned with their own fears to watch you or care what you are doing.

How to Search

Search for an appealing woman who appears to be approachable. How approachable a given woman seems will depend on your experience and level of skill. For most men, it is easiest to approach a woman who is alone. A woman with other women is more difficult, and approaching a woman who is with a man is the most difficult. Until you become skilled at this process, it may not seem easy to approach any woman.

There are two ways to search. You can circulate through the crowd, or you can position yourself somewhere and watch women pass by. Standing near the entrance is good because you can check out the women as they arrive. Another good place to stand is near a busy "choke" point where women will pass near you.

When you first arrive, search by circulating through the crowd to see who is there. After that, you can alternate between searching by standing and watching women pass by and searching by circulating through the crowd. If one of these methods seems more effective for a given event, it's okay to use it exclusively. The only hard and fast rule is to not stand around talking with your friends. That is not an effective search strategy. And don't ever think that you can stop searching because you have seen all the women there. New women will be arriving all the time, or a woman may have been hidden from view when you searched earlier.

Steps 2 and 3—Get Near and Break the Ice

Once you have selected a woman, you must get near enough to speak. In some situations you can get near first and then wait a few minutes before speaking to her. In other situations you will have to walk directly up to a woman and speak to her immediately. Here is how to handle four typical situations at a mixer.

Situation No. 1—A Woman Who Is Standing in a Crowd With No Companion

Most men think that a woman in this situation is the easiest to approach. Because she is in a crowd, you can work your way through it and then stand near her without her noticing your approach. When you get near, you can stand there awhile without speaking. Then, when the moment seems right, you can casually say something to break the ice, such as:

"Is this place usually this busy?"

"Do you know the name of this band?"

Just getting near can help. Once you are near her, you might notice something that you can use as an icebreaker. That happened to Alex at a singles mixer:

I was standing near a woman, trying to think of something to say, when a young man with purple hair walked by. His hair was sticking straight out from his head like he had stuck his finger in a light socket. When the woman looked at this guy's hair, I turned to her and said, "Would you like the name of his barber?" That's all it took to get a conversation started.

If Alex had been across the room from this woman trying to think of something to say, he would have missed this chance for a good spontaneous opener. The man with purple hair provided him with an excuse to say something. As Alex can tell you, it pays to get near a woman as soon as you realize that you want to meet her.

Situation No. 2—A Woman Standing Away From the Crowd and Alone

You can't walk up to a woman who is standing all alone and not say something to break the ice. You have to use an icebreaker as soon as you get near. In this situation you don't have the option of standing next to her while you think of something to say. Therefore, have an icebreaker ready as you approach her. One of the following straightforward openers would work:

"Hi, my name's Steve. What's yours?"

"You look professional tonight. Do you work nearby?"

This gutsy, straightforward approach will become less intimidating after you try it a few times and get a few positive reactions.

Women frequently go to singles mixers with a friend or friends. Once there, they often stand facing one another, with their backs to the men, and carry on what appears to be an engrossing conversation, as if they haven't seen one another in years (they probably work together and see each other every day). In most cases these women are really there hoping to meet men, but the meat market atmosphere makes them nervous. The closed conversation circle is their way of reacting. When a man thinks about trying to meet a woman who is in such a group, he often has one or more of the following concerns:

- ♦ He feels that interrupting their conversation might seem rude.
- ♦ He doesn't know how to start and sustain a conversation with a group of women.
- ♦ He wonders how he is going to let one woman know he is interested in her and not her friends.
- ♦ He is concerned about asking a woman for a date in front of her friends.
- ♦ He is reluctant to hurt the feelings of the other women by showing no interest in them.

For the above reasons, most men don't like to meet a woman who is with other women; therefore, it is to your advantage to learn how. If you do, you won't have much competition. We will explain how to meet a woman in two situations: a woman with one other woman, and a woman with several other women.

Situation No. 3—A Woman Who Is With One Other Woman

You will often see a woman you want to meet talking with another woman. If they are apart from a crowd, you will need to say something as soon as you get near. One of the following icebreakers would be good.

"Hi! How are you two doing tonight?"

"So did you two get caught in the traffic on Broadway?"

If they are in a crowded area, you can stand close by and wait for a momentary break in their conversation before saying something. When there is a break, you could say:

"So how was your day at the office? Any dramas or tragedies?"

"What do you two think of this band?"

After you use your icebreaker, they will usually turn toward you to talk. At this point, stand somewhat closer to the woman you want to meet. This gives them their first clue about whom you are interested in. As the three of you talk, gradually direct more of your questions to the woman you find appealing. After a little conversation among the three of you, you can begin to get a conversation going that is just with the woman you like. You do this by the way you ask follow-up questions. For example, you could ask the general question, "What do you two do for a living?" When her friend says she is a C.P.A. and the woman you are trying to meet says she is in sales, look at your selected woman and reply, "Sales! How interesting. What do you sell?" You can then start to meet your conversation goals by talking to the woman you are interested in. Sometimes the other woman will excuse herself and leave you two alone. If the other woman doesn't leave, don't be deterred. Carry on with the rest of the steps. It may be more difficult for you to ask for a date in front of another woman, but you have much to gain and little to lose.

Situation No. 4—A Woman Who Is With Two Or More Women

Sometimes the woman you want to meet will be in a conversation with several other women. When they are in a group conversation, approaching them is a bit more difficult than when a woman is with just one friend because they're likely standing in a closed circle. To break into their circle and become part of the conversation, stand just outside the circle and near the woman you want to meet, and show an interest in what they are saying. The women will be aware of your presence and will usually open their circle to include you in the conversation. When this happens, use your icebreaker. Say something that applies to the whole group. For example, you could say:

"Hi! Do you all work together?"

"You all are adventuresome to be out on such a stormy night."

After a little conversation with the entire group, gradually focus your attention on the woman you want to meet by directing your questions just to her. When there are three or more women in a group, the other women will often sense what is going on and start up another conversation among themselves. You are then free to achieve your conversation goals.

The above techniques for getting near and starting conversations with women at singles mixers are valid. You may approach a situation exactly as we described, however, and the situation may shape up differently. That is to be expected. The important thing to remember is that it is *possible* to meet women alone or in groups at singles mixers. When you see a difficult situation, such as a woman in a group, accept it as a challenge and use your ingenuity to overcome the obstacles. After you accept a few of these challenges you will learn that you can survive no matter how the situation turns out. You will also learn that on occasion, you will get a date when you didn't think you could.

Step 4—Continue the Conversation

If you are dancing with a woman at a singles dance and you can't think of anything to say for a minute or so, it won't seem awkward because you can still enjoy dancing together in silence. If you are talking to a woman who is on the exercise machine next to yours at a health club and the conversation slows down, it won't be awkward because you can continue working out until you think of something else to say. If you have just started a conversation with a woman at a singles mixer and you can't think of anything else to say, it immediately gets awkward, however, because at a singles mixer the conversation is the primary activity. There is no handy diversion to help you out when the conversation dies. To keep your conversations from stalling, ask questions and make comments that will help you achieve your conversation goals. When you do that, the conversation will flow naturally, and you will get valuable information to help you decide if the woman is right for you.

Conversation Goal No. 1—Get Insurance

Mike has just met Helen at a singles mixer, and they are ten minutes into an interesting conversation. Mike is planning to ask her for a date before the evening is over. Suddenly Helen's girlfriend rushes up to her and says, "I just called the sitter—Bobby is sick. I have to get home right away." Helen turns to Mike and says, "We came in the same car—I have to go." She pauses and looks hopefully at Mike for a moment. Mike is overwhelmed by the sudden change of events and doesn't have time to gather his thoughts. Helen says, " 'Bye," and she is gone—out of Mike's life, probably forever. Because Mike didn't get insurance, there is no way for him to contact her in the future.

Interruptions such as this are common at singles mixers; therefore, it's important to get insurance early in the conversation. When, for any reason, you don't get a chance to close, insurance will give you a second chance at a date.

Insurance (the woman's name and enough information about her work to enable you to phone her there) is easy to get at a singles mixer because mixers are typically held right after work. "What kind of work do you do?" and "Do you work nearby?" are natural questions to ask.

Here is how Brent obtained insurance from a woman who worked at a large company.

Jane had introduced herself using only her first name. I wanted to be sure I could get in touch with her again in case I wasn't able to get her number, so I asked her questions about her work. The conversation went like this:

BRENT: "What do you do?"

JANE: "I'm an executive assistant."

BRENT: "Which company?"

JANE: "I work for City Gas and Electric."

BRENT: "What level is your boss?"

JANE: "He's a vice president."

BRENT: "What's his name? Maybe I know him."

JANE: "Abramowitz."

BRENT: "How do you spell that?"

JANE: "A-B-R-A-M-O-W-I-T-Z."

BRENT: "Was that A-B-R-A-M-O-W-I-T-Z ?"

JANE: "That's right."

BRENT: "I don't think I know anyone named Abramowitz."

We continued talking for a while, and eventually I asked Jane if I could call her sometime. She said she didn't want to give out her number, but would take mine and call me instead. I haven't had much luck depending on women to call me, but in this case I wasn't worried, because if Jane didn't call, I felt that I had enough information to reach her at work. I would call City Gas and Electric and say to the operator, "I'd like to speak to Jane—Vice President Abramowitz's assistant."

The next day Jane did call, so I didn't need to use the insurance. But when she called, the first thing she said was, "You know, I got your card out and laid it on the bed and left the room. When I came back in to call you, my cat was chewing on your card. I could barely make out your number."

Jane probably didn't realize that the cat could have eaten the entire card, and it wouldn't have mattered because she would have still heard from Brent. Brent had insurance that was good enough to reach her, even at a big company like City Gas and Electric. That's why you get insurance—for unexpected situations.

Tip: *If a woman won't give you her number and asks for yours instead, one way to emphasize that you really want to hear from her is to bet her dinner out that she won't call. She will probably feel that she can't lose because she has your number and you don't have hers. What she probably doesn't realize is that you have insurance and can reach her at work. If she doesn't call within a day or so, call her at work and say, "This is Jim. We met at the singles mixer. I think you owe me dinner. Remember?"*

Conversation Goal No. 2—Qualify Her

The cocktail-party atmosphere at a singles mixer makes it easy to talk long enough to really get acquainted. The questions you ask to find out if a woman meets your requirements will keep the conversation flowing and give you useful information. Unlike meeting in some other situations, there are no particular questions that need to be asked at a singles mixer. You are free to focus the conversation on the topics that will give you important information about her.

Tip: *It is usually best to avoid talking about your divorce, your ex, or your past girlfriends. It is definitely in bad taste to gaze around the room looking at other women.*

Conversation Goal No. 3—Extend Your Time Together

Although extending your time together is an option, it is not of particular importance at a singles mixer. If you were standing in a shopping mall talking to a woman, extending your time by getting a cup of coffee together would give you a chance to talk in a more comfortable setting. Standing at a mixer having a long conversation is not awkward because it is what everybody is doing (or wishes he was doing). Although extending your time at a singles mixer is not of great necessity, it does have some value. Your suggestion to do something else together tells a woman that you are interested in her. Her acceptance tells you that she is interested in you. If there is an art display in the lobby, ask her whether she has seen it. If there is a buffet table, suggest getting a bite to eat together. You could also ask her if she would like to go to the restaurant next door where the two of you could talk over coffee. Doing something else together starts the transition from a conversation between two strangers to something more romantic.

Step 5—Close

At a singles mixer you don't have to talk all evening before asking a woman for a date. After twenty minutes or so of conversation the two of you will probably have decided whether you want to go out. If she doesn't want to go out with you, the sooner you find out the better, because you can then spend your time looking for another woman. Talking to a woman who isn't interested in you is a waste of time.

For the most part, closing at a mixer is like closing anywhere else. You can either get her phone number or you can arrange a date first and then get her number. As always, it is good to suggest an activity that you know she enjoys. Therefore, during your conversation make it a point to find out what she likes to do in her spare time.

Sometimes you will be faced with asking a woman out in front of her friends. Many men avoid doing this, thinking that they will have a big audience when they get shot down. When a woman is with friends, however, you don't have many options. If you want to ask her out, you are probably going to have to do it with her friends watching. After you have done this a few times, you will start to get over your apprehension.

A singles mixer is a perfect place to ask for a date for that evening because the woman may have come straight from work without having had dinner. If so, invite her to join you at a nearby restaurant. If you are going to drive to the restaurant separately, exchange phone numbers before you go just in case something unexpected happens that keeps either of you from getting there (such as a car breakdown or someone getting lost). If you don't have the dinner option because the woman has already eaten, suggest going somewhere to listen to music or to a dance spot.

Ron, a friend of ours who learned our Five-Step technique, seemed to do everything right the night he met Pam.

Pam and I met at a singles mixer. It was a mob scene that night. I had gotten tired of forcing my way through the crowd, so I found a place to stand where the people were threading their way through the crowd, single-file. After a few minutes, three women who appeared to be together walked in front of me. One of them was wearing a tight, red knit dress that caught my eye. As she squeezed by, she saw me looking at her, and with a sly smile she said, "Well, did I pass inspection?" I thought her outrageous remark needed an outrageous reply, so I said, "What did you expect? This is a meat market, you know." She laughed and we started talking. When I asked her what she liked to do for fun, she said country dancing was her passion. When I heard this, I asked her if she would like to leave and go do some country dancing at Pistol Willie's. She said it sounded like fun, and she left me for a moment while she told her girlfriends that she was leaving to go dancing with me. We traded business cards before we drove to Pistol Willie's in separate cars.

Ron didn't waste any time once he decided that he liked Pam. A little conversation, an invitation to go dancing, and they were on the way to their first date.

If you ask a woman for a date and get a refusal, start over with the search step. But what if you ask her out for another night and she agrees to go? In that case you can either get her number and leave for the evening or get her number and continue talking with her. But there is one thing that you should never do, and that is take her number and then leave her while you hustle other women. That is definitely in bad taste, and could easily cost you your date with her.

13

How to Meet a Woman While Riding a Bike

When we encourage the men in our class to try bike riding as a way to meet women, most are skeptical. Some say they ride a lot, but have never met a woman that way. We tell these skeptics that it isn't a matter of going out riding and waiting for an accidental meeting to occur; it's a matter of having the skill and putting forth the effort to make it happen.

One student told the class about his buddy Arnie, who knows how to meet women on the bike paths:

Early one Saturday morning last summer Arnie stopped by my house on his bike and announced that he was heading for the bike paths to try to meet a woman. I didn't think he had much of a chance. I figured that if he rode often enough, he might meet a woman by accident, but if he expected to meet someone that particular day, I was sure he was going to be disappointed.

About five that afternoon, Arnie stopped by again. When I asked him how he had done, he said, "In eight hours I saw five women I was interested in meeting, approached each one, talked to each one, and asked each of them for her phone number. I now have five numbers I didn't have this morning. It was an amazing day. I have approached five women in eight hours before, but this is the first time I have ever gotten five phone numbers."

Needless to say, after hearing Arnie's story, the next Saturday I dusted off my bike and headed for the bike path. I rode for two hours and didn't see a woman who would be easy to meet. Discouraged, I gave up and rode home. When I told Arnie what had happened, he was not sympathetic. He said, "You only rode for two hours? Lots of times I ride the whole morning and don't see anyone. You gave up too soon. Let's go out tomorrow and see what we can do together."

The next day we rode a bike path that goes by some big condo developments and then ends up at a park downtown. Arnie said a lot of women from the condos ride this path. When we came to the top of a hill, Arnie stopped and surveyed the scene in every direction. Then he said, "See those two women with bikes on that street corner? Let's go meet them." It seemed ridiculous to go after them because they were about a quarter mile away, but that didn't seem to bother Arnie. He took off like a shot. I followed along, hanging back a bit because I was embarrassed. I couldn't image that this was going to look like an accidental meeting.

We raced along the bike path, across a bridge, over some railroad tracks, and stopped next to the two women. Without hesitating, Arnie said, "Nice day for a ride, isn't it?" They responded in a friendly way and Arnie continued talking, asking them about their bikes and where they were headed. After talking with them for about five minutes, Arnie suggested that we all ride over to a bagel shop on the next block where we could sit outside and have a snack. The girls agreed to go. As we were about to separate after having our bagels, Arnie arranged for us to meet them that evening at the park to listen to an outdoor concert.

While Arnie and I were riding home, I said, "You made that look so easy. How did you learn to meet women on the bike path?" Arnie replied, "I picked it up kind of by accident. I would occasionally speak to women on the bike path, and I usually got a friendly reply. Eventually I realized that I could go out riding with the sole purpose of meeting a woman. So one day I did and

I got a date. Once you hit pay dirt a few times, you gain a lot of confidence and become highly motivated."

Advantages of Meeting a Woman While Riding a Bike
The greatest advantage of a bike is the mobility and versatility it gives you. You have the mobility to search parks, bike paths, city streets, and beaches. You have the versatility to approach women who are walking, jogging, riding a bike, sunbathing, or just sitting on a bench reading.

When you see a woman in evening clothes under the soft lights of a singles place, a lot is hidden. On a bike path you get to see women in the daylight, and usually in sportswear, so you get a pretty good idea of what they look like.

There is also a more subtle advantage: Most women say a man who approaches on a bike seems less threatening than one who approaches on foot. Consequently, you have a better chance of success on a bike compared to being on foot.

Disadvantages of Meeting a Woman While Riding a Bike
You are limited to good weather and daylight hours. Not many women are in a park or on a bike path when it's cold or dark. Therefore, if you live where winters are cold, bike riding shouldn't be your only method for meeting women.

THE FIVE STEPS WHILE RIDING A BIKE

Step 1—Search
The power of a bike is most apparent on the search step, because on a bike, you can search a large territory. Bike paths, city streets, parks, beaches, and other public areas are all open to you. Bike paths and parks near condos and apartments may have more single women than paths and parks near single-family homes. Get a bike path map and plan a route that will cover some parks, beaches, downtown walking areas, and other places where women will be sunbathing, walking, jogging, in-line skating, or riding bikes.

A second way to search is to find a place where a lot of people pass by, then get off your bike, wait, and watch. Look for appealing women who don't have a male companion and who are not wearing a wedding ring.

Tip: *If you are going to wait and watch, choose an inconspicuous place where you can see women go by, but where they won't notice you. If a woman sees you sitting there watching her, and then notices that you are following her, she might become apprehensive.*

Step 2—Get Near

How you get near depends on what the woman is doing. Here are the three common situations you might face on a bike:

1. She Is Going Away From You

This is the easiest situation. When the woman is walking, jogging, or biking in front of you, catch up with her. When you get close, go just a little faster than she. As you slowly ride by, you will be close enough to speak.

2. She Is Coming Toward You

This is the most common situation, and for many men, the most difficult. When you are riding along a bike path and you see an appealing woman riding or jogging toward you, all you have to do is one simple, but possibly embarrassing, maneuver—after she passes, make a U-turn. Most students protest, "But she'll know what I'm doing." They're right; she probably will know what you're doing, but it really doesn't matter. If she's interested in meeting you, she'll be glad that you made a U-turn, and she might be impressed by your nerve. If she's not interested, it hasn't hurt you. She wouldn't have gone out with you anyway.

Jim told us about the day he learned that he had nothing to lose, and everything to gain, simply by turning around:

On the first warm day last spring, I left work early to take a bike ride and try to meet a woman. About twenty minutes into the ride a woman came riding toward me. When she rode past,

I knew I wanted to meet her, but I hesitated because I had two problems: I felt embarrassed about turning around, and she was wearing a headset. A headset is a serious deterrent to a casual hello. But then I thought, "She is really good-looking! I have to meet her." I turned around and rode after her.

As I rode up beside her, out of breath from the chase, but trying to be casual and calm, I shouted, "Nice day, isn't it?" She gave me a perplexed look (I really hate headsets!). Feeling like a fool, I shouted the greeting again. This time she finally got the idea that I wanted to talk with her. She struggled with the headset controls. Again I shouted a greeting, and the third time was the charm. "Yes, it's a great day!" she said with a big smile. What a relief. I got through to her and her response was friendly, even enthusiastic.

After about ten minutes of riding and talking, I asked her if she would like to do some "off pavement" riding at an area I knew. She agreed, and we set off for a ride which I knew would take at least thirty minutes. Now I could relax and talk to her, knowing she wouldn't dart off the bike path at any moment and head home. At the end of the ride I asked her to go riding with me another time. She agreed and gave me her number. Making the U-turn and outshouting the headset turned out to be worth it.

The "U-turn" approach may not be easy, but it is often required. Most of the women you will see will be riding toward you.

3. She Is Stationary

This situation can be somewhat difficult because the woman will probably be watching as you make your approach. For example, if you are riding in a park and you see a woman sunbathing in the middle of a large grassy area, there will be no way for you to just appear beside her as if it were a chance encounter. Since there is no alternative, get your nerve up and do what you must do to meet her—walk right up to her and start a conversation. Keep in mind, however, that many women feel less apprehensive when approached by a man on a bike than when approached by a man on foot without a bike. For this reason, if you are going to approach a woman you see at the beach or reading on a grassy area, walk with your bike or ride your bike up to her. Don't park it somewhere and then walk up to her.

Step 3—Break the Ice

Just before you break the ice you will either be approaching a woman from behind who is moving away from you or approaching one who is stationary.

1. Icebreakers to Use When Approaching a Woman From Behind

As you ride up beside her, smile and say something like, "Nice day, isn't it?" or "Having a good ride?" or "Having a good run today?" These are reasonable icebreakers, but almost any opener will do. What you are doing is testing the water to see if she is open to some conversation. Therefore, your opener is not critical, but her reaction to it is.

Reactions can vary greatly. She may express fear, annoyance, suspicion, surprise, or sheer delight at having a man speak to her. Unfortunately, there is no way to tell in advance which reaction she is going to have. The woman who looks the least friendly may be the one who reacts most favorably. If you speak to several women on a ride, you will probably get a wide range of reactions.

Tip: There is a nonverbal method to see if a woman on a bike wants to talk with you. After a few minutes of conversation, ride several feet in front of her (when riding on a bike path it is often necessary to ride single file to make room for oncoming bikes). Once in front of her, hold a steady speed. If she catches up, she is interested. If she doesn't, she is probably not interested.

If a woman does not react with an obviously friendly response, continue talking, because a few more comments may be necessary to establish how open she is to your company. Have a few follow-up remarks in mind, such as, "Jogging far today?" or "So is this your usual way of getting exercise?" If she begins to show some interest, continue talking. If she doesn't respond or if she seems frightened or annoyed, respect her feelings and ride on. Don't keep talking to her when she is bothered by your presence. Leave with a friendly, "Have a nice day."

2. Icebreakers to Use When Approaching a Woman Who Is Stationary:

While the icebreaker "Nice day, isn't it?" is perfectly okay to use to test the water when you are riding past a woman, when approaching a woman who is stationary, there are better icebreakers to use. When the woman is stationary, use an icebreaker that will lead to further conversation. For example:

She is standing beside her mountain bike: "That's a great-looking bike. Is it new?"

She is feeding ducks: "The ducks are hungry today. What are you feeding them?"

She is watching a soccer game: "Do you know which teams are playing?"

It's a good idea to envision the various situations you might encounter on your bike and plan icebreakers that will be appropriate for each situation. Sometimes, however, you will have to come up with a spontaneous icebreaker, as Reed discovered:

I was riding my bike around the park when I noticed an attractive woman sitting alone on a blanket reading a book. I wanted to meet her, but how was I to make contact? It would take a direct approach across fifty yards of open grass to get near her. I was very uncomfortable with the thought of such an obvious approach, and I couldn't think of anything to say that would sound reasonable. After three more times around the park, I finally thought of something to say. Knowing what I was going to say helped me get up the nerve to ride across the grass directly toward her. I got off my bike a few yards away, walked up to her with the bike, and said, "Is that a good book you're reading?" She looked at me suspiciously and said, "Yes, it is good." It was a definitely neutral, almost negative, response. It was an awkward situation. I almost moved on, but after such a brief conversation, that would be as embarrassing as hanging around. Groping for a follow-up I said, "What's it about?" That helped some. As we talked about the book, she became friendlier and more open to having company, so I sat down to continue the conversation. After about thirty minutes, I asked her if she'd like to go out sometime. She accepted and I got her phone number.

It was touch and go for Reed during the first few minutes. He almost gave up and left after her first not-so-friendly response. A neutral or even a negative response is fairly common in such situations, however. A woman may be surprised when you speak to her, and it might take a few minutes before she starts responding in a friendly way. Sometimes it's a tough call whether to hang around and continue talking or to give up.

Step 4—Continue the Conversation

Once you have a conversation going you can focus on getting insurance, qualifying her, and extending your time together. When you are talking with a woman who is riding a bike, it's important to get insurance early because at any moment she could say, "Here's my turnoff, nice talking with you," and she's gone. If you don't have insurance, you will probably never see her again, but with insurance, you still have a chance. When the woman is stationary or walking, getting insurance quickly is less critical because if she decides to leave, you might still have time to close.

When speaking to a woman who is moving (walking, jogging, or riding a bike) make an offer to extend your time together early in the conversation. If she accepts your offer to do something together, you will know how much time you will have with her before you have to close. Extending your time is important if she is moving because she could depart suddenly. After about ten minutes of friendly conversation, make an offer to extend your time together. Here are some examples:

"I'm going to ride around Green Lake. Want to go with me?"

"I was thinking of stopping for some lunch. Want to join me?"

"Want to stop and get something to drink at that refreshment stand?"

If she agrees, you have a fairly good idea of how much longer you have to talk with her. If she says no, her refusal may give you a clue as to how much longer you have to talk. For instance, she might say, "I'd like to, but I need to get home. One more lap around the park and I have to leave." This is valuable information. You now know that you must close during the next lap.

Larry extended his time with a woman he met on a recent ride, with excellent results:

I was riding my bike one day, trying to meet a woman, when I noticed a young woman in front of me running with her dog. I slowed down to evaluate the situation. She was short, thin, and had very nice legs—definitely appealing. Her dog was off the leash; this gave me an idea for an icebreaker. As I rode up next to her, I said, "Does your dog bite?" She replied, "Oh no— he's friendly." "What kind of dog is it?" I continued. She replied in a friendly way, so I kept talking. After about ten minutes I said, "I'm going downtown for some breakfast. Would you like to join me?" She said, "Sure—but I have to take my dog home first and change clothes. Come on back to my house. I'll change, get my bike, and we can ride downtown to eat." Some women have no fear of strangers.

It was good that Larry offered to extend their time together when he did, because he learned later that she was near the turn-around point in her run when he made the offer to get breakfast. If she had suddenly said, "I'm turning around here. See you later," before he had suggested breakfast, chances are he would have not reacted quickly enough to close. He probably would have just kept on riding.

Another way to find out how much time you have is to ask a few simple questions. For example:

"How long are you running today?"

"Are you riding all the way to City Park?"

"This is a nice day. I'm spending all day outside. How about you?"

The answers to such questions might tell you how much time you have before you must close. Once you know, you can relax, do some qualifying, enjoy the conversation, and be thinking of what kind of date you will suggest if and when you close.

Step 5—Close

Other than *when* to close, closing during a biking encounter has no unique problems. If she is on a bike, an offer to go for a bike ride would be good. If you found out that she likes tennis, an offer for a game of tennis would be good. The date you suggest probably doesn't matter much; any safe date would be okay.

The Five Steps can help you meet a woman on a bike path, just as they can in other face-to-face meeting situations. In addition to knowing how to apply the Five Steps, however, be ready to put in the time. A thirty-minute bike ride around a park may not be sufficient. Many hours of riding is usually what it takes.

❦14❦

How to Meet a Woman at a Singles Bar

*T*he techniques presented in this chapter are based on the assumption that you know how to "touch dance." That's the kind of dancing where the man leads and the woman follows. Country-western (Texas two-step and three-step), Latin (cha-cha, rumba, and tango), and ballroom dances (waltz and fox-trot) are examples of touch dancing. Singles bars (also referred to as clubs, nightclubs, dance spots, and night spots) that feature this kind of dancing are recommended because it's easy to talk with a woman while touch dancing. Bars that feature "freestyle" dancing (where the man and woman stand apart and dance separately) are less desirable because it's difficult to carry on a conversation while freestyle dancing. In a singles bar that doesn't have dancing, use the techniques presented in chapter 13, "How to Meet a Woman at a Singles Mixer."

Advantages of a Singles Bar
♦ Singles bars are open almost every night of the week, and they stay open late. If you don't have any other activity scheduled, there are always women in the clubs. If you have gone to another event earlier and it is now ten o'clock at night, you can drop by a club to see who is there.

♦ At a singles bar there is a built-in reason to start a conversation. What could be easier than saying, "Would you like to dance?"

♦ A singles bar is a good place to practice meeting women because it is perfectly acceptable for you to dance and talk with different women all night. Where else could you get so much practice in one evening?

Disadvantages of a Singles Bar

♦ The secondhand cigarette smoke may be hazardous to your health.

♦ Some women are especially wary of men they meet in a singles bar. These women may be reluctant to go out with you simply because of where you met.

♦ Some women who go to singles bars discover that they get a lot of male attention. Sometimes this makes them very selective.

♦ It's difficult to tell a woman's age in a dimly lit bar.

♦ The "meat market" atmosphere, where everyone is on display and looking everyone else over, makes some people uncomfortable. This is mostly a matter of an individual's perception, however. Some people are extremely conscious of it, while others are oblivious to it.

How to Get Used to the Singles Bar Atmosphere

Despite the bad reputation of singles bars, there are decent women in them every night of the week hoping to meet someone special. Most single women go to a singles bar at least once. If you avoid singles bars, you are cutting off one possible avenue for meeting single women. If you haven't tried the singles bars, however, it is only fair to warn you that you might be overwhelmed by the whole scene on your first visit.

If you are going to give the singles bars a try, plan on going at least three times before you make a decision about whether or not they will work for you. Any new place takes some getting used to, but a dark, noisy singles bar that is crowded with strangers can be especially intimidating, so don't give up too soon. It almost always gets easier after each visit. After a while, you might even start to enjoy it.

On your first trip to a singles bar you might ask a few women to dance and get turned down. Don't get discouraged—it happens to all of us. Rejection comes with the territory in singles bars (and other places as well). Few of us are so handsome that every woman we desire automatically desires us in return.

Tip: *If you see a woman who starts her evening off by giving several men a big hug, she is a club regular. If she is attractive and has been coming into that singles bar often enough to be on a hugging basis with the men regulars, she has had many opportunities to get into a relationship and, for whatever reason, has chosen not to. It is possible that she is holding out for the right guy, and you may be just the man she is looking for, but don't get your hopes up too high. If you ask a bar regular for a date and she doesn't accept, don't take it too hard. You have just added your name to a long list of men who have received similar rejections.*

How to Choose a Singles Bar

Different singles bars attract different clientele. Do some research on the bars to find out where your type of woman is most likely to be. To find out where the singles bars are in your area:

♦ Look in the entertainment section of your newspaper under "Dancing," "Night Life," or "Clubs."

♦ Ask your friends.

♦ Keep on the lookout as you drive around town.

Trial and error is the best way to find out which places appeal to you. Some singles bars appeal to a younger crowd and some to an older crowd. Some feature one kind of music and some another kind. When you find a singles bar that seems right for you, ask the men and women there where else they go. They might be able to tell you about other bars that are similar.

Tip: If a club is close to your home, you are likely to meet a woman who lives nearby. If you drive a long distance to a club, you are more likely to meet a woman who lives far away.

Best Nights of the Week in Singles Bars

After you have been in a bar a few times you will notice that some nights of the week are dead and on other nights the place is really jumping. You may also notice that there is a night when one bar is slow, while a bar down the street is crowded. You can speed up the process of finding out which nights are best in a bar by asking the bartenders, waitresses, and other patrons.

If a single woman with young children would be acceptable to you, keep the typical custody arrangement in mind when deciding which nights to go. On weeknights you will see mostly young women with no children and older women whose children are grown. The women with young children are normally home with their kids. Under many custody arrangements, the father takes the children on weekends, often picking them up on Saturday. With this visitation schedule, a single mother often has Saturday nights free, and that is the night that she is most likely to be in the clubs. In addition to single mothers, many other single women who don't get out during the week go to the clubs on Saturday night, while many single fathers are home with their kids. You may like the ratio that you see on Saturday night.

You older singles may remember a time when there was a stigma attached to going out on Saturday night without a date. That stigma no longer exists. Saturday night has become an important night for going out to meet someone.

Here are some generalizations about the different nights of the week in the singles bars. Individual bars may vary from this pattern because of ladies' night specials (no cover charge or special drink prices) or because of special entertainment features.

Sunday: Some singles bars close on Sunday night. Others have a teen night with no alcohol served. If the bar is open to its regular customers, it is probably the slowest night of the week.

Monday: A slow night.

Tuesday, Wednesday, Thursday: May be lively or slow, depending on bar promotions and the whims of the crowd. Bars generally get busier as the week progresses. There will be mostly young women with no children and older women whose children are grown.

Friday: A busy night. Pretty much the same type of women as during the week, only more of them. The bars get busy early on Friday as people stop in after work to unwind.

Saturday: The busiest night. You will see many women who weren't there during the week. Because fewer clubs have two-for-one drink specials (i.e., "twofers") or free buffets on Saturday night, the activity may start later in the evening.

Best Time of Night to Go to a Singles Bar

Early in the evening singles bars often feature twofers and free (or inexpensive) buffets. These clubs get busy early as patrons flock in after work for the bargains. When people come in later for dancing, they are pleased to see that there is already plenty of activity. Many women who go to a singles bar for the after-work buffet will leave early and be replaced by women who come out later for the dancing. You will see the greatest variety of women by going for the buffet and staying for the dancing.

How Long to Stay in One Singles Bar

If you live where there are several singles bars, staying in one club for the entire evening may not be the best strategy. If you have approached all the women you desire in one club, the only reason you would stay in that club would be to see who comes in later. While you are waiting the entire evening for a clientele turnover of perhaps 50 percent where you are, however, another club would have 100 percent different women. It may be more effective for you to take a few minutes and drive to another club. Going to several clubs may increase your chances of success.

This technique of going to several clubs is especially effective during the week when the clubs are slow. On Friday or Saturday night the clubs are usually packed, with women coming and going in large numbers all evening. Under these conditions it may not be as effective to go from club to club. Whether to stay in a club or move on is a matter of judgment.

What to Drink

If you are going to several singles bars in one evening, you might be concerned about the amount of alcohol you will consume. You don't have to drink alcohol at every bar, however, or any of them. You have several nonalcoholic options:

♦ Order coffee, soft drinks, or bottled mineral water.
♦ Order juice (orange juice and Bloody Mary mix are usually available).
♦ Order nonalcoholic beer.
♦ Order a glass of water (tipping the waitress or bartender when you order water is courteous).
♦ Don't order anything.

Disadvantages of Going With a Friend

Many men are in the habit of going to the singles bars with a buddy. If you do this, consider its effectiveness. Here are some of the disadvantages of going with a friend:

♦ If he can't go out, you will stay home too.
♦ You will have a tendency to talk to him instead of actively trying to meet a woman.
♦ If you are ready to move on to another club and your friend wants to stay, you have a conflict. If you stay to keep him happy, you might be wasting your time.
♦ When you go with your buddy you are increasing the competition. Hard feelings may develop between the two of you if you like the same woman.

When we ask the men in our class why they go out looking for a woman with a friend, they typically reply, "It's okay for us because we like different kinds of women." We wonder if that's really true, or if they are using their buddy as a security blanket. If you and your buddy have learned to meet women as a team, however, and if your technique is effective, by all means continue to go out together.

Age in Singles Bars

If you are approaching middle age or are into it in a major way, there is a good news–bad news story for you. The good news is that the dim lights in the singles bars are very kind. Your wrinkles, that slight puffiness in your face, and that hint of gray in your hair will not be obvious. You will look years younger than you are, whether you want to or not. The soft lights are a double-edged sword, however—it is also difficult to guess the age of a woman in a singles bar. Some men automatically add ten years to their best guess.

If it is important for you to know the woman's age, you can ask her questions to get the information you need. There is a problem, though; it doesn't seem to be good form to directly ask a woman her age. You could ask her what year she graduated from high school and assume that she was eighteen at the time, but we don't recommend this technique because it is a very poorly disguised way of asking for her age. There are some questions that you can weave into the conversation that are not quite so blatant, however. For example, you can get an estimate of a woman's age by asking her if she has any children. If she does, you can inquire about their ages. As a rough rule of thumb, if the woman didn't go to college, she probably had her first child when she was between nineteen and twenty-three. If she graduated from college, she probably had her first child between twenty-three and twenty-seven. You may miss it by a few years using this technique, but you will usually get in the ballpark.

If the woman is divorced, you can back into her age by first asking her how long she has been divorced and then asking her how long she was married. These are both topics that divorced singles talk about frequently and easily. Next you can casually ask, "How young were you when you got married?" You now have all the numbers you need to calculate her age. If she has been married and divorced several times, you may need to do the math on a table napkin.

THE FIVE STEPS IN A SINGLES BAR

Step 1—Search

When you enter a club, the first thing you should do is look around for the best place to sit, right? Wrong! The first thing to do is to start searching for a woman to meet, and when you search, never sit down. There is nothing you are going to do that requires you to be seated. You are there to act and make things happen, not to rest your feet. The sooner you get busy searching, the better. Delaying action usually makes you more hesitant and less likely to act.

Here is how to do an effective search in a singles bar:

- When you first enter, walk through the entire club and see who is there.
- If there are no women there you want to meet, stand near the entrance and watch who comes in.
- Periodically walk through the crowd again. An appealing woman may have been in the restroom, dancing, or otherwise hidden from view when you did your first walking search.

Carl learned an important lesson one evening in a singles bar.

I had been in Cadillac's (a singles bar that plays oldies but goodies) for about half an hour, having a beer, and trying to get the nerve up to ask a woman to dance, when my friend Doug came in. He saw me sitting there, so he came over to say hello. After a couple of minutes, he said he had to get to work, and I watched him make a pass through the entire bar. I sat there with my beer. Then he went right up to one of the women and asked her to dance. They danced, and I sat there with my beer. After a few dances, he walked her back to her seat and stayed and talked to her for about five minutes. I sat there with my beer. Then I saw them exchange phone numbers, and he came back over to me and said he had a date.

I learned a valuable lesson that night. When you walk into

a singles bar, swing into action right away. When you sit down with your beer, you don't get your nerve up; somehow sitting makes it harder to get into action, not easier. In the time it took me to have a beer, Doug got a date.

Doug seemed to know how to meet a woman in a singles bar. He did everything right, including beginning his search of the bar quickly and not wasting a lot of time with his friend Carl.

Tip: If you are going to get a drink in a singles bar, get it from the bartender, not a waitress. If you order a drink from a waitress, she is going to expect you to stay in one spot until she returns with your drink, possibly five minutes later. You don't need to lose this much search time rooted to one spot.

Steps 2 and 3—Get Near and Break the Ice

In nonsingles places such as parks and shopping malls you have to find creative ways to do Steps 2 and 3. You have to think of some way to get near, and you have to come up with an icebreaker. In a dance spot, Steps 2 and 3 require no creativity because they are done as a set routine. You walk right up to a woman and say, "Would you like to dance?" That's the beauty of meeting women in a dance spot: You have a built-in reason for approaching a woman, and you have a ready-made icebreaker.

Tip: You may see a woman and her friends working their way through the crowd to find a place to sit or stand. You could remain where you are, standing on your tiptoes, straining to see where she goes. A more effective technique is to fall in behind the group when they pass in front of you, and work your way through the crowd with them. That way, when they stop, you are already standing near the woman you want to meet. You are ready to start a conversation or ask her to dance.

Step 4—Continue the Conversation

Once you are dancing with a woman, it is easy to carry on a conversation. Don't get so swept up in the fun of dancing that you forget to ask her qualifying questions. Because many women are wary of men they meet in a dance club, during your conversation make an extra effort to establish that you are a safe, stable, and pleasant man.

Conversation Goal No. 1—Get Insurance

Getting insurance (her name and enough information about her work to be able to reach her there) is not as important in a dance bar as in some other places. When dancing with a woman you are usually safe from interruption for the length of at least one song, and probably several. Interruptions do occur, however. The disc jockey may call an intermission for a contest or some other form of entertainment, or your partner may not like the next dance number. Because you can't be sure how long you will be dancing with a woman, it is a good idea to always get insurance early in the conversation. Then, if you fail to close for any reason, you can reach her later at her work.

Gordon got insurance at a singles bar one evening, and it paid off:

I met this gorgeous young lady in a singles bar that had the loudest music I have ever heard. I don't know why they do that, it makes it so hard to talk. I danced with her for a few songs, but we weren't able to talk because it was that stand-apart-and-wiggle kind of dancing.

After we walked off the dance floor, I leaned over and yelled in her ear, asking for her name and where she worked. She yelled back, "I'm Becky. I work as a receptionist for a home security firm." I then yelled, "What is the company's name? She called out, "Fairbrother Security." I asked her to repeat it to be sure I had it right.

I wanted to ask Becky out to lunch, but I couldn't bring myself to scream out, "Would you like to go to lunch this week?" Asking for a date is hard enough without having to scream it out. So I just said good-bye and thanked her for the dance. I immediately borrowed a pen from a waitress and wrote on a paper napkin: *Becky, Receptionist, Fairbrother Security.*

I looked up Fairbrother Security in the phone book when I got home that night, and called the next morning. When Becky answered the phone, I said, "This is Gordon. We danced last night—remember? I had on a blue shirt." Becky responded with a surprised, "How did you get my number?" I laughed and said, "You told me where you worked."

After she had gotten over her initial surprise, she sounded happy that I had called. When I asked her if she could meet me for lunch the next day, she said that she would like to go, but she wondered if it would be okay if she brought her girlfriend along. I didn't know if she had already made plans to have lunch with her girlfriend or if she was just playing it safe, but it didn't matter to me if her girlfriend went along; I was glad to have a date with Becky.

Conversation Goal No. 2—Qualify Her

Dancing is great for qualifying. You can count on several minutes of uninterrupted conversation, and if you ask the right questions, in two or three dances you should be able to find out if a woman meets your most important requirements. In a fairly short time you can usually find out enough to know whether you want to ask her out.

Conversation Goal No. 3—Extend Your Time Together

There is usually not much need to extend your time with a woman you are getting to know in a dance place. In many other situations, such as meeting a woman at a lecture, a shopping mall, or an airport, a suggestion to have a cup of coffee together provides for a smooth transition from a casual encounter to the start of a romantic relationship. In a singles dance bar, this transition is not necessary, because everyone knows that people go to singles bars to find romance. On occasion, however, there may be situations where it is useful to extend your time with a woman in a singles bar. For example, if it is so loud in the bar that you can hardly hear each other talk or if you want to get her away from another man, a suggestion to leave to get a cup of coffee and some dessert could be useful. For such situations, extending your time together can be an important part of your strategy for getting a date.

Step 5—Close

A singles bar is one of the easiest places in which to close because everyone knows what is going on—most of the men are there to meet women, and most of the women are there to meet men. In this environment women will seldom be caught off guard when you ask for a date. In addition, when you are dancing with a woman, your conversation is private, and that makes it easier to ask for a date.

One way to close is to wait until a dance number is over and then ask her for a date as you walk her off the dance floor. You can suggest a specific activity or simply say, "Could I call you?" If you get a negative response, simply thank her for the dance. If you get an acceptance, walk her back to her seat where you can get her phone number and work out the details of the date.

It's best to suggest a date that she will consider safe, because many women are concerned about the type of man they are meeting in a bar. You may want to suggest lunch or some other daytime activity in a busy public place. When suggesting a date say, "I can meet you there or pick you up, whichever you prefer." If she wants to meet you there, it's critical that you exchange phone numbers so that you can reach each other in case a change of plans becomes necessary.

How Soon to Close

If you like the woman, and she has been dancing and talking with you for several dances, it's time to close. You don't have to dance with her all evening or sit at her table and buy her drinks before you close. She has probably already decided whether she wants to go out with you, and there is usually little to be gained by waiting to ask her out. There is a downside to waiting too—you could be wasting your time if she is not interested in you. To avoid wasting time on someone who won't go out with you, ask for a date relatively soon. Asking for a date after one dance is a little quick. Four or five dances, however, should be sufficient for the two of you to learn enough about each other to decide if you want a date.

There is a feeling among many inexperienced men that the proper thing to do is to spend the entire evening with the woman before finally asking for a date. Ken felt that way until he had an experience that changed his mind forever.

I was in a country-western dance bar, and at about nine o'clock in the evening I spotted a woman sitting at a table with two girlfriends. I asked her if she would like to dance, and she said that she didn't know how to dance western. When I told her that I could teach her, she accepted my offer. From nine until midnight I gave her dance lessons, bought her drinks, and sat at her table talking with her and her friends. I was excited about how well I was doing with her, and I began to think that I had found a girlfriend. At midnight I told her that I had to go, and asked her if we could go out dancing again sometime. She replied, "I don't date. I'm a realtor. I work odd hours, and I'm raising my son. I don't have time to date."

That was the last time I ever spent three hours with a woman before asking for a date. That woman knew at nine o'clock that she didn't date. I didn't find out until midnight. I entertained her the entire evening, gave her dance lessons, and bought her drinks. I felt used. Now I never spend hours with a woman before asking her out, and I seldom buy anyone a drink. I don't think a woman is impressed by the fact that I can afford a couple of bucks for a drink.

A few women want to know a man fairly well before accepting a date. If you ask one of these women out within ten minutes, she is not likely to accept; however, you have no way of knowing how long you will have to talk with her before she will accept. Will she accept after thirty minutes? An hour? Two hours? Or perhaps she won't go out with you after any length of conversation. How long to wait before closing is always a judgment call.

A Refusal to Dance is Not Necessarily a Rejection

If you ask a woman to dance and she turns you down, you need to interpret her response. Not all refusals to dance mean the same thing. If she looks you in the eye and says, "No, thanks," this usually means, "No, I don't want to dance with you now or in the foreseeable future." In this case you should give up and move on to find a woman who is interested in dancing with you. There are many other responses a woman may give that are open to interpretation, however. Here are some of the responses you might get when you ask a woman to dance, along with what her response could possibly mean.

"Come back later," "Maybe later," and "Can I take a rain check?" could mean:

- ♦ I'd like to dance with you, but my girlfriend and I are talking. I'd feel rude leaving her right now.
- ♦ I just ordered a drink and should be here when the waitress brings it.
- ♦ The dance floor is too empty. I'd feel conspicuous dancing right now.
- ♦ I have been dancing a long time and need a break.
- ♦ I just lit a cigarette and want to enjoy it for a few minutes.

"I never dance until I've had two drinks" could mean:

- ♦ I'm not comfortable with this whole singles scene. I need a few drinks to relax.

"Not this number" could mean:

- ♦ I don't know how to dance to this music.

"I don't know how to dance slow dances" could mean:

- ♦ I don't dance slow dances. I had a bad experience on the dance floor—sometimes men want more than a dance.

"I don't dance fast dances" could mean:

- ♦ I can't do the fast dances, but would like you to ask me to dance if they play a slow song.

"I don't dance" could mean:

♦ I can't dance.

Steve is a friend of ours who is a club regular and an excellent dancer. We asked Steve what he thought women meant when they said, "Maybe later," and Steve replied, "They mean, get lost, sucker!" When asked if he ever went back later to ask again, Steve said, "Never!" Steve's reaction is typical of what most men feel when they get a refusal. Yet a certain percentage of the time the woman only meant that now was not a good time, but she would like to dance later. You can increase your chances by going back a second time. Try to satisfy her request for a fast song, a slow song, a dance at a later time, or whatever. Sometimes you will get a second refusal, and sometimes you will get an eager acceptance.

Tip: *When you ask a woman to dance, watch her eyes. If she glances at the dance floor and then turns you down, often the problem is not you, it's the dance floor. A woman who is uncertain about her dancing ability will want the dance floor to be fairly crowded before she gives it a try. The thought that everyone will be watching her may be making her feel uncomfortable.*

If you see a woman give this quick glance at the dance floor, or if she says that she can't dance or can't dance to that music, you have a perfect opportunity to help her while you get to know her. She probably wants to get out on the dance floor and join the fun, but she is not confident about her dancing ability. If you know how to dance to the music being played, tell her that the dance is easy and you can help her learn. Often just a few words of encouragement are all that it takes to convince a reluctant woman to take the plunge. View her refusal as an opportunity, not a rejection.

In those situations where you ask a woman to dance and you get turned down, you always have the option of forgetting about the dancing and instead trying to continue the conversation. Asking,

"Do you want to dance?" can just be an easy way to get a conversation started. A negative response to the dance request doesn't necessarily mean that you have to walk away.

Tip: *When you ask a woman if she would like to dance, she may point to her companion and say, "No, but my friend here would." This can create an awkward situation for everyone involved. You probably saw her companion when you searched the place, and if you had wanted to dance with her, she would have been the one you asked. When this situation arises, you can avoid rejecting the companion by dutifully dancing with her. If you aren't interested in her, however, you are wasting your time. Therefore, when this occurs, don't let your eyes follow the woman's finger when she points to her companion. Simply keep your eyes riveted on the woman you have asked to dance and say, "Thanks anyway," and walk away. Because you have not looked at her friend, her friend does not feel as if she has been rejected because of her looks.*

ADVANCED TECHNIQUES

How to Meet a Woman Who Is With Another Man

You may have been in a club and seen an appealing woman, but passed her by because she was with another man. If you did, you were just doing what the majority of men would do in a similar situation. You may also have been passing up a golden opportunity. Women are sometimes in singles bars with a man with whom they have no romantic connection. There are many reasons why a woman may be in the company of another man. For example, some women want to get out to meet men, but are afraid to go to bars alone. They might ask their brother, their uncle, or a platonic male friend to accompany them.

When a woman is with a man, how she is interacting with him can help you read the true situation. For example, when a man and woman are seated at a table, leaning toward each other, touching, and gazing into each other's eyes, you would be an absolute fool to ask her to dance. But if they are sitting with chairs well apart and looking uninterested in one another, they may not be romantically involved. Clues to look for when a woman is sitting with a man are a bored look on her face and her foot bouncing in time with the music. This may be her way of saying that she wants to dance and she wishes some other man would ask her. If her companion is not dancing with her, he may be there only as a platonic escort. Such a woman may be quite receptive to your request for a dance.

Another common situation that you will see is a man sitting at a table with two or more women. Again, watch the interaction between the man and the woman you're interested in to make your decision about the level of involvement. A student in one of our classes said she went to a dance once and sat at a table all evening with her girlfriend and her girlfriend's date. She said that she wasn't asked to dance a single time, she wasn't happy about it, and she wondered what was wrong with men. What is wrong is most men don't have the sophistication to read such situations. If you do, you may be asking a woman to dance who has been waiting a long time to be approached.

You may not feel comfortable asking a woman to dance who is in the company of another man, and some men we know think that it is unwise. Obviously, you have to read the situation carefully and weigh your desire to meet the woman against the possibility that you are going to anger the man. If you are reluctant to ask a woman to dance in the presence of a male companion, wait until she makes a trip to the rest room and ask her before she gets back to her seat. Or wait until the man goes to the rest room and ask her while he's gone.

How to Meet a Woman by Rescuing Her

How can you tell that a woman needs to be rescued? There are two situations that are common. Sometimes you will see a man take a seat next to a woman on a bar stool and try to get a conversation going. If you see that their conversation has run out of steam, be aware that the ensuing silence can be awkward for the woman. So if there's not much conversation between them, her eyes are wandering, and she looks bored, free the woman from the awkward silence by asking her to dance. She may be relieved that you rescued her.

Another situation that you might see is one of a man standing beside a woman who is seated at the bar, and he is talking endlessly. Some men do this as a way to sort of guard a woman they have just met. Such a man appears to feel that as long as he is standing beside her talking, other men are not likely to approach her. She may want other men to approach, however, and she may be annoyed that the endless talker is keeping them away. If you observe that the woman is not doing much of the talking, or she looks annoyed or bored, you have an opportunity to rescue her. When there is just the slightest pause in the conversation, approach from the side opposite the man and quickly ask the woman for a dance. On the dance floor she might say, "I'm *so* glad you got me away from him. He was a total bore and I didn't know how to get rid of him."

Randy is a friend of ours who loves to dance. He gets most of his dates in dance clubs. He was bragging to us once about how he met a woman who was with another man. Here's Randy's story:

A very striking woman came into the club on the arm of a man. There was something about the situation that made me feel she wasn't romantically involved with him. She was attractive and well-dressed, while he had on jeans, and his most noticeable feature was his beer belly. The man was obviously excited to be in her company—he kept touching her and standing with his arm around her. He seemed almost giddy to have such a prize for the evening.

I wanted to dance with this woman so I could ask her out, but he never left her side. I decided to wait until one of them went to the rest room and ask her then. A half hour later I saw her headed in that direction, finally alone. I zipped up along-side her and said, "Are you spoken for this evening?" She replied, "Oh, I guess I have to stay with him. We went to high school together. He was passing through town, so he called me to see if we could meet for a drink."

I knew I only had a few seconds before she would return to him, so I just came right out and asked her if we could go out dancing sometime. She replied, "I will be here with my girlfriend on Thursday. If you can make it then, I'd like to dance with you."

She did show up on Thursday, and after dancing together for a good part of the night, I made a date to meet her for lunch.

Randy was obviously not new at this business of meeting women. He was perceptive enough to suspect that this attractive woman with her unlikely male companion might be available. He realized that his only chance to meet her would be when either she or her companion went to the rest room. That worked like a charm, and after finding out that she didn't have much time to chat, he got right down to business and asked her out.

What Not To Do?

Paul is one of our students who hasn't been on the singles scene long enough to have learned Randy's advanced techniques. As a matter of fact, Paul sometimes still makes a mess of things. Here is his story about a situation that he could have handled better:

I was in a singles bar when I saw a woman I wanted to get to know. It took a long time for me to get my nerve up, but I finally asked her to dance. She accepted, and after we had danced for a little while, I asked her if I could buy her a drink. She smiled and nodded, so I found a table and we waited for the waitress to come by. But the waitress looked busy, so I went up to the bar to get our drinks. There was a crowd around the bar, and I didn't get our drinks right away.

When I got back to the table, Jenny was dancing with another man. I sat down with the drinks and waited for her to return, but she just kept dancing with that man. She seemed to know him, and it looked as if they were having some kind of argument. I was getting plenty irritated about the situation. Then Jenny's beast of a girlfriend sat down at the table. She said, "Is this Jenny's drink?" I said it was, and she proceeded to drink it. Since I was already mad as hell about Jenny dancing so long with that guy, when her friend started drinking the drink I had bought Jenny, it was more than I could handle. I reached across the table and took the drink away from her, downed it in one gulp, and stomped out of the place.

Paul's disaster illustrates several important points about getting a date in a singles bar. Paul felt that he needed to buy Jenny a drink and sit at a table and talk for a while before asking her out. He could have done all the talking he needed to do while he had her in his arms on the dance floor. When you delay asking for a date, things can go wrong, as Paul found out.

Paul's second mistake was to leave Jenny alone in this club full of hungry men and go to the bar to get a drink. A woman sitting alone at a table is fair game in these places. If you need to buy a woman a drink, wait until the waitress comes to your table. When you leave a woman alone, you give other men opportunities.

Paul's final mistake was to lose his temper. When Jenny's girlfriend started drinking the drink he had bought for Jenny, Paul lost control. If Paul had just remained calm, he could have still pursued a date with Jenny. He could have continued to sit at the table with Jenny's girlfriend, talking with her about Jenny and the man she was with. He may have been able to get insurance on Jenny through her girlfriend. He may also have learned what the romantic connection was between Jenny and the man she was dancing with. Or Paul could have just been patient and waited for Jenny to return. After all, Jenny and her dance partner seemed to be in a fight of sorts, which was probably a good sign for Paul.

You now know the basics of getting a date in a singles bar that has dancing. If you have an idea of what to do to meet a woman in the singles bar environment, you will be head and shoulders above most of the men there. Now that you have the basics, the next thing to do is to find the best bars and go to them until you get used to all the noise and congestion. When you go, practice what you have learned in this chapter. If you know what to do and have the skill to do it, singles bars can be gold mines of opportunity.

❧15❧

How to Meet a Woman at the Beach

$\mathcal{I}$n many ways the beach is a perfect place to meet a woman. Everywhere you look there are scantily clad women. Yet you see so many men alone, or in groups of two or three, not doing a thing to meet them. Many of these men come to the beach without a woman in their life, spend the day watching and wishing, and leave at the end of the day, still alone and lonely.

That is the typical situation at the beach; it's a great place to meet a woman, yet surprisingly few contacts are made. The reason is simple: The women are waiting for men to approach, but most of the single men are afraid. To meet a woman at the beach, you have to do more than just lie in the sun or talk to your buddies—you have to take action to make it happen. Apply the Five Steps in the beach environment and your chances of getting a date will increase dramatically.

Advantages of the Beach

♦ You get to see what the women really look like. Compared with seeing a fully clothed woman in the dim lights of a singles bar, seeing a woman in a bikini in broad daylight gives you a much more accurate picture.

♦ You may meet women at the beach who don't go out much to meet men. Either they don't like the meat-market atmosphere of singles meeting places or they are single mothers who have a hard time getting out. In either case, since they don't make themselves accessible to men, they may not get much attention, and that could make them very open to meeting you.

♦ Few men know how to meet women at the beach. If you learn how, you will have little competition.

Disadvantages of the Beach

♦ You can meet women at the beach only during daylight hours and in warm weather. If you live where the winters are cold, you shouldn't make the beach your only way of meeting women.

♦ Since the beach is not just for singles, many of the women there could be married or involved. If you happen to ask a woman out who is in a relationship, in most cases she will be flattered. The worst that will happen is you will get rejected. So what?

THE FIVE STEPS AT THE BEACH

At the beach you will see women standing in line at the concession stand, lying on their beach towels, cooling off in the water, and strolling along the water's edge. Other women might be playing volleyball or throwing a Frisbee with a girlfriend. All this activity means there are many different ways to apply the Five Steps.

Step 1—Search

Although it is important to do the search step at the beach, most men either don't do it or don't do it well. They follow a routine of sitting or lying on a beach towel and occasionally getting up to cool off in the water. Much of their time is spent on their towel, rooted in one spot. These men search by looking over the top of a book (through dark sunglasses). Sitting or lying on a beach towel is not an effective way to search.

The dynamic environment of a beach calls for an active search where you assess the meeting possibilities in an organized manner. For example, when you are searching you might see a desirable woman in a situation that makes you feel that it would be hopeless to try to meet her. Farther down the beach you might see an equally desirable woman in a much easier meeting situation. You should locate several women you would like to meet and then consider how easy it would be to approach each of them. You will then be ready to evaluate both the women and their approachability, and select one to approach first.

Search by walking some length of the beach. If you walk along the water's edge, occasionally walk through the middle of the crowd, some distance back from the water's edge, so you can also see the women who are there. Pass by the concession stand occasionally to see who is in line. If you have searched the crowd without success, position yourself where you can see new women arriving. After ten minutes or so, do another walking search to see if you missed any women. A woman might have been in the rest room or otherwise out of view when you did your first search.

It's important to search actively, and this means moving about. You are looking for a good meeting opportunity as well as a desirable woman. Meeting opportunities at a beach will be changing constantly. You can't keep track of changing conditions along the length of the beach by lying on your towel.

There is another good reason to do an active search. If you are lying on your beach towel and see a woman you want to meet, in order to meet her you have to get up and start moving. Now this may not sound like a big deal, but when the fear of rejection is combined with inertia, you just might decide to stay where you are. On the other hand, if you are walking down the beach, actively searching, and you see a desirable woman ahead, you will keep moving in her direction quite normally—the fear of rejection won't keep you frozen in one spot. Moving about can help put you in the mood for taking action. Lying in the sun can put you in the mood for sleeping.

Steps 2 and 3–Get Near and Break the Ice

Women at the beach will be engaged in a variety of activities. The technique you use to get near and what you say to break the ice can depend on what she is doing. Therefore, steps 2 and 3 will be examined together for some of the most common beach situations.

How to Get Near When She Is on a Beach Towel

If you are bold, you can walk directly up to a woman who is sitting or lying on her beach towel and immediately speak to her. If this is more than you can handle, however, you can use the indirect technique of placing your towel within speaking distance of her. The more crowded the beach, the closer you will be able to get without feeling intrusive.

If the beach is not crowded, you might find it awkward to place your towel near enough to her to easily start a conversation. If so, place your towel a comfortable distance from her, but in a position where she is between you and the water. With your towel in that position you will have numerous chances to speak as you pass by on your way to and from the water.

How to Break the Ice When She Is on a Beach Towel

Before you even go to the beach, you should plan a few icebreakers that will work at the beach, no matter what the woman is doing. Then when you see a woman in a particular situation, you have the option of using one of your planned icebreakers or a spontaneous icebreaker that pertains to that woman or that particular situation.

Having a few planned icebreakers gives you something to fall back on in case you can't come up with something better. For example, if the woman is lying on her beach towel, you could use a planned icebreaker such as:

"Aren't we having a great summer?"

"Have you been in the water yet?"

"Are you here on vacation?"

Or you might be able to think of a spontaneous icebreaker that pertains to her, the place, or the situation you are in. For example:

She has the pattern of a bow on her sunburned back: "I'll bet your other bathing suit ties in back with a bow."

"Did you get to see the volleyball finals earlier?"

"How long do you think we have before that thundercloud rolls in?"

How to Get Near When She Is in the Water

If the woman looks as if she has gone into the water for a quick dip, position yourself by the water's edge where you will be able to speak to her when she comes out. If she is floating on an air mattress or inner tube and it looks as if she will be there awhile, go out in the water and get near her.

How to Break the Ice When She Is in the Water

When you get near her, you can use one of your planned icebreakers, or a spontaneous icebreaker such as:

"The water's really cold. Are you getting used to it?"

She's on a giant inner tube: "Where in the world did you find such a big inner tube?"

How to Get Near When She Is at the Concession Stand

If you have been hanging around the concession stand and you see an appealing woman get in line, get in line right behind her. The concession stand is a good place to meet a woman because you have an excuse for getting near.

How to Break the Ice When She Is at the Concession Stand

Once you are in line behind her, you can use your planned icebreaker or say something about the line of people or the food. For example:

"This is a long line. It looks like I'm not the only one who's thirsty."

"How do they make those curly fries?"

How to Get Near and Break the Ice When She Is Walking Away From You

When she is in front of you and walking away from you, catch up with her. Then slowly pass by her and test the waters to see if she is friendly and open to some conversation. Make a cheerful comment, such as, "Nice day, isn't it?" and watch her reaction. If you get a cheerful response, follow up with another question to continue the conversation such as, "How far are you walking?" If after two or three comments you don't get a friendly reaction, she probably doesn't want your company and it is best to leave with, "Have a nice day."

How to Get Near and Break the Ice When She Is Walking Toward You

If you and the woman are walking toward each other, stop walking when she gets near and get ready to use an icebreaker. In this situation, an icebreaker that is just a pleasantry won't do, because she will probably respond with a similar pleasantry as she walks away. For example, if you say, "Nice day, isn't it?" she will probably reply, "Yes it is," as she walks on by. Your icebreaker in this situation must be something that will increase the chance that she will stop to respond to you. We call these icebreakers that make women stop and talk "grabbers."

Stan learned about grabbers when he was at the beach one day.

I was standing by the edge of the water when I saw four young women in bikinis walking toward me. I made eye contact with one at some distance, and I think she noticed that. When she got close, she gave me a big smile and said, "Hi! How are you today?" I was caught off guard by her outgoing nature. I only got out a weak "Fine" as she passed by. I felt that she wanted to meet me, so I spent some time trying to get close to her again. But soon she and her friends were all wrapped up in a volleyball game and I never was able to meet her.

Later that day I saw how another man handled the same situation that I had muffed. A group of women were walking toward him, and when they were close, he blurted out, "Hey girls—what's happening?" The girls all stopped to talk with him. At first, I thought "Hey girls—what's happening?" sounded pretty stupid, but then it sank in that he knew how to get the girls to stop and talk—something I had failed to do.

Every once in a while you will come across a woman who is actively trying to meet a man. For heaven's sake help her. When that young lady in a bikini asked Stan how he was today, he should have replied, "Fine," followed immediately by a grabber, such as, "Where are you guys headed?"

Step 4—Continue the Conversation

A beach is an easy place to sustain a conversation because women there usually have time to kill. If a woman has been lying on a beach towel for a long time, she might be bored and appreciate some conversation. Once you are in a conversation with a woman at a beach, try to achieve your conversation goals.

Conversation Goal No. 1—Get Insurance

At the beach it is not as important to get insurance early in the conversation as it is in other situations, such as in a supermarket or on a bike path, where the woman may depart with little notice. At the beach you usually have time to talk for a while, and you would probably have plenty of warning that she is getting ready to leave. Even though it is not critical that you get insurance early in the conversation at the beach, it is still important to get it at some time during the conversation. Be sure to get at least her first name, and weave into the conversation questions about where she works and what she does there. Then, if for some reason you are unable to close, you probably have all the information you need to reach her by phone when she is at work.

Conversation Goal No. 2—Qualify Her

Ask questions during the conversation to see if she meets your requirements. And while you are at it, find out what activities she enjoys so you can suggest one of them as a first date.

Conversation Goal No. 3—Extend Your Time Together

Extending your time together is especially useful if you are in a situation where it is awkward to carry on a lengthy conversation. If you are sitting in the sand next to a woman while carrying on a conversation, finding a way to extend your time together is probably not critical. On the other hand, if you are standing by the water's edge or in the water, talking, an extended conversation may get awkward. In these situations a suggestion to get something from the refreshment stand or to go sit on the beach and talk might create a more comfortable setting for an extended conversation. If she agrees to your suggestion, you have a clue that she is interested in you.

Step 5—Close

At the beach, as at other nonsingles places, how soon to close is a judgment call. Close too soon and she may think that you are a skilled "beach hustler" who approaches women at the beach all the time. You may be just such a hustler, but it is best if she thinks your meeting was an unplanned, romantic encounter. On the other hand, if you wait a long time to close and then she turns you down, you have wasted a lot of time—time you could have used trying to meet a woman who would be interested in going out with you.

As a general rule, a conversation of about thirty minutes before you close would probably be appropriate. Closing after a five-to-ten-minute conversation would probably be too soon at a beach (although it would be perfectly acceptable in singles meeting places, such as in a dance spot). Talking for an hour or more is taking a chance that you are wasting too much time.

What kind of date activity should you suggest when you close? A woman who is at the beach without a man may be facing a lonely evening. You might get a positive response by suggesting the two of you have dinner that evening. Offer something specific. Tell her that you know a place that has the best pizza in town or a place where you can eat out on a deck overlooking the water. Give her the option of meeting you there or of your picking her up, whichever she is most comfortable with. You might also suggest an activity that she has expressed an interest in during your conversation, or you could suggest meeting for lunch the next day.

Tip: *When it is time to get her number, it may not be cool to pull a pencil and paper out of your bathing suit pocket—that looks a little too professional. Make sure you have a pencil and a scrap of paper in your beach bag, but rummage around in the bag for a while, acting as if you are not sure that you have a pencil and paper.*

If you ask a woman for a date and she turns you down, say that you enjoyed talking with her, give her a cheerful good-bye, and start over with the search step. If she accepts your offer, you then have a choice. You can spend a few more minutes talking with her and then make an excuse to leave by saying something like, "I had better get going. I have some errands to run. I enjoyed talking with you." Or, if you have the time, and she seems comfortable talking with you, continue the conversation for as long as you want. Whatever you do, don't excuse yourself and then try to meet another woman—that's bad form.

In summary, meeting a woman at the beach is an active process where you move around in search mode, continually trying to create meeting situations. If you want to meet the woman on a beach towel near yours, meet her within the first few minutes or give up. Don't lie there all day trying to get up the nerve to meet that one woman. Get up off your towel and swing into action. See what other opportunities there are up and down the beach.

At a beach there are many creative techniques you can use to meet women. If you are at a lake and you own a boat, have it pulled up nearby and offer women rides or a chance to water ski. If you are going with a buddy, take a Nerf ball or a Frisbee and arrange for it to conveniently land exactly where you want. Or you can take a camera and ask the woman to take your picture so you can send it to your mother. Then offer to take her picture and say you will send it to her. Of course, to do that you will have to get her name and address.

Adrian used a sand castle as a way to meet a woman at the beach. Here is what he did:

> I was walking along the water at the reservoir one day, trying to find a woman I wanted to meet, when I spotted a woman building a sand castle. She was using a "dribble method" where she would let the wet sand dribble from her hand onto the top of the castle. It had an interesting decorative effect. I had just passed some young men who were using buckets to build a huge castle. I used the sand castles to open a conversation with her, saying, "Their castle is a lot bigger than yours." She replied, "Yes, but mine is more beautiful." I asked her which was more important, size or beauty, and she replied, "In sand castles, beauty is everything."
>
> Since she had a big smile on her face and no wedding ring, I sat down in the sand beside her so we could talk. When I introduced myself, she said, "My name is Melody—like in the song, 'A Pretty Girl is Like a Melody.' "
>
> I spent the better part of an hour getting to know her, and then I asked if I could call her sometime. She agreed and gave me her number.

Adrian did a good job. He wasn't lying on his beach towel dreaming of meeting a woman. He was walking the beach, actively looking for opportunities. When he saw a woman he wanted to meet, he made it happen by using the spontaneous icebreaker, "Their sand castle is a lot bigger than yours." That got a conversation started, and he carried it on until he had Melody's phone number.

It may seem strange to go to a beach just to meet a woman, but it can pay off. Next time you are at home on a warm day wishing you had a girlfriend, think of the many women at the beach who might be very pleased to meet you. Go there and give it a try. You will either wind up with a date or you will wind up better at meeting women than you were before because of the practice you got.

How to Meet
a Woman at Airports
and on Airplanes

*a*ir travel offers many good, but usually overlooked, meeting opportunities. Once you know how to apply the Five Steps in that environment, flying will no longer be boring; it will be yet another exciting way to meet women. Whenever you fly on business, there will be opportunities to meet a woman at the airport and on the plane. If she lives in the city where you are going, you might get a dinner companion while you are there. If she lives in *your* city, there is the possibility of a relationship with her. Even if you don't get a date, you might have someone interesting to talk with on the flight. It's a win-win-win situation if ever there was one. All that is required is a little know-how and some nerve. So don't take a flight somewhere and then go out looking for a woman (or spend a lonely night in your hotel)—look while you are flying. Maybe you will end up with a date before you arrive.

Advantages of Air Travel
♦ Air travel provides an opportunity to meet women in your everyday life.

♦ Most women feel comfortable talking to strangers at airports and on airplanes.

♦ There are often long, uninterrupted time periods when you can carry on conversations.

♦ There's little or no competition because few men try to meet women while traveling.

♦ A bombshell who won't give you the time of day at a singles event might be glad to talk to you on an airplane.

Disadvantages of Air Travel

♦ You may meet a woman who lives far away.

♦ At a singles event most women are available. On an airplane there's less of a chance.

When traveling by air you will see women in many different situations. They may be shopping in an airport store, eating in one of the restaurants, waiting in the baggage claim area or on a taxi line, or riding the train between terminals. The Five Steps can be used to meet a woman in any of these situations. We will show you how to customize the Five Steps for two typical situations where you might have time to kill—in the waiting area before boarding and on the airplane.

THE FIVE STEPS BEFORE BOARDING

Step 1—Search

If you get to the boarding area early, say thirty minutes before flight time, you will be able to check out nearly every woman on your flight. Watch the women checking in to see if their husbands or boyfriends are seeing them off. If a woman is alone, look for a wedding ring.

Step 2—Get Near

In waiting areas people sit and stand wherever they want and nobody pays much attention, so when you get near a woman, it will probably not be obvious to her. A woman you want to meet will often be in one of the following situations: waiting in line to check in, waiting for boarding to start, or waiting in line to board. To get near, do whatever she is doing. If she gets in line to check in, get in line behind her (if you have already checked in, get in line behind her to reconfirm your seat assignment). If she is waiting for boarding to start, try to stand or sit next to her. If all else fails, get in line behind her to board the plane and try to have a few minutes of conversation to at least make her aware of your presence.

Tip: *This is a long shot, but when you check in you can always ask, "Could you put me next to a nice-looking woman?" Sometimes it works.*

Step 3—Break the Ice

It's easy to strike up a conversation in a waiting area because most of the people there are just killing time. Here are some icebreakers you can plan on using to get a conversation started:

"Do you live in [the departing city or destination city]?"

"Are you headed home?"

(The above two questions are good because they let you know where she lives.)

"Is the plane supposed to be on time?"

"So what's the weather like in [destination city]?"

"Is [destination city] your final stop or are you flying on?"

"What do you think of [airline you are traveling on]?

Spontaneous questions or comments about such things as the weather, the airport, her clothes, a book she's reading, or her laptop computer also make good icebreakers.

Here is what happened when Rick did the search, get near, and break the ice steps while in an airport waiting area:

I was sitting there waiting for the line at the check-in counter to get shorter when this slender, attractive woman got in line. I quickly got in line behind her and said, "So where are you headed?" That started a short, but lively, conversation. When we got to the counter I said, "Let's get seats together. Is that okay?" She agreed, so I asked the ticket agent to seat us together. We had a very nice conversation during the two-hour flight. I ended up going out with an aerobics instructor.

Step 4—Continue the Conversation

When you are talking with a woman in a waiting area, qualify her early in the conversation by finding out where she lives. Then, if you are still interested in her, get insurance (her name and where she works) as soon as possible, because in a waiting area you never know how long your conversation is going to last. You might think that you have plenty of time to get to know her, when suddenly she departs to make a phone call or visit the ladies' room.

Step 5—Close

If you have talked to a woman for a comfortable length of time (perhaps ten to twenty minutes) and you are still interested, close before you board. If she lives in your city, arrange a date when both of you will be in town. If the two of you are flying to the same city, arrange to go out with her there.

If boarding is about to begin and you don't think that you have talked long enough to ask her out, suggest sitting together on the plane. You could say, "If there's room on the plane, would you like to sit together and continue our conversation?" If she agrees, find seats together. If you can't get seats together, don't give up; there may be an opportunity to talk to her again after landing.

Tip: *View a delayed flight as an opportunity to meet a woman. No one is going anywhere, and you have a lot of time to strike up a conversation.*

John turned a long delay into an exciting night out. Here is what happened:

I was stranded once at London's Heathrow Airport, along with hundreds of other people. It was noon, and all flights, including mine to New York, had been canceled. We weren't going to be able to get out until the next day. Some people were sitting around reading or talking, others were napping on the floor. I decided that I didn't want to sit around the airport when there was a big, fascinating city just a subway ride away.

I searched through the crowd for an unattached, appealing woman whom I could invite to go into London to have dinner with me. After a long search, I saw a beautiful young woman sitting alone on the floor. I was in my mid-forties then, and she appeared to be in her early twenties. This big age difference, and her striking good looks, made the thought of approaching her especially frightening. But I took a deep breath, walked over to her, and said, "Where are you going?" She said, "Los Angeles. Where are you going?" and gave me a big smile. After talking with her for a few minutes I could sense that she was open to company, so I sat on the floor next to her. Her name was Sherry, and, as I found out later, she was twenty-three-years old.

After we talked for about ten minutes, I said, "Would you like to get a cup of coffee or tea?" She gladly agreed, and we had a nice conversation over tea, exchanging travel stories. I was definitely interested in her, and much to my surprise, she seemed interested in me. After we had talked over tea for about an hour, I said, "Would you be interested in taking the tube to London? We could hit a few pubs and grab some dinner." Again, she seemed pleased with the invitation.

We had to get rid of our luggage before going downtown, so we got in the baggage storage line, along with hundreds of others who apparently had the same idea. Thirty minutes later this three-hundred-foot line had moved five feet. My excitement over spending an evening with this gorgeous young woman began to turn into frustration. Then I had an idea. I excused myself and phoned a small hotel I knew in central

London. I asked the desk clerk, "Do you have any rooms for tonight?" He replied, "We have two left. One with twin beds and one with a double bed." I said, "I'd like to reserve the one with the double bed. Let me check with my partner and I'll call back in ten minutes."

Back in the baggage storage line I made a gutsy offer to Sherry. I said, "We'll never get downtown at this rate. I just called a hotel in London and they have one room left, a double. We could leave our luggage at the hotel and go out for the night, and then spend the night in the hotel. No sex expected." I really didn't think she would agree, but at this point, what did I have to lose? She thought for a moment and then said, "Yes, that would be fine." Elated, I called the hotel back and confirmed our reservations.

After dropping off our luggage at the hotel, we wandered around London, visited a few pubs, had dinner, and slept together in the hotel (without sex, in case you are wondering). It was a great night out.

John's experience not only shows that meeting women at airports is possible, it also shows how "extending your time" can lead to a surprisingly good outcome. John made three separate offers to extend his time with Sherry:

1. An Offer to Get Tea

This was appropriate after ten minutes of conversation between two strangers at an airport. When Sherry accepted his offer to get tea, John knew that she was alone and interested in some company.

2. An Offer to Go Into London to Hit the Pubs and Have Dinner

This would probably not have been appropriate after ten minutes of conversation, but after an hour talking over tea, she liked the idea.

3. An Offer to Spend the Night Together

John made this offer sooner than is usually appropriate, but the situation forced him to do something to avoid spending a boring night at the airport.

Continually extending your time with a woman is a great technique in situations where the woman is not expecting a romantic encounter, such as at an airport. In a singles bar a request for a date after a ten-minute conversation would be fine. In an airport or other nonsingles place, an offer to get a cup of coffee is more appropriate after a ten minute conversation than is a request for a date.

THE FIVE STEPS ON AN AIRPLANE

If you are not successful meeting a woman in the waiting area, don't give up. There will be additional opportunities once you are on the plane. Once you are flying, before you settle down with your laptop or book, see if there are any opportunities to meet a woman.

Step 1—Search

As soon as the seat belt light goes off, and before the drink carts block the aisle, walk to the front of the plane. Then slowly walk to the back of the plane, noting where any appealing women are sitting. Look for wedding rings, and notice which women have an empty seat beside them.

Step 2—Get Near

If there is more than one acceptable woman, approach the ones toward the back of the plane first. If you start at the front, the woman in the back may be put off when you approach her because she has seen you talking to other women.

Step 3—Break the Ice

It is easiest to break the ice when the woman has an aisle seat because she is close and easy to talk to. Once you are standing next to her seat, kneel down and ask, "Would you like some conversation on the way to [the destination city]?" If she is agreeable, sit next to her. If not, go on to the next woman.

If she has a window seat and the center seat is vacant, it is more difficult, but still doable. Just sit down and say, "Excuse me. Would you like some company? If you don't, it's okay." Most women are surprised by such a direct approach, but not frightened, because they are in a safe place. If she agrees, you have a chance to talk with her for the rest of the flight. If she doesn't want company, thank her and move on.

Step 4—Continue a Conversation

Once you are seated next to a woman, it is easy to continue the conversation. You have a known amount of time to talk to her, and you will not be interrupted. Use this time to find out where she lives and whether she is available. If you are still interested, use the conversation to continue qualifying her. Since you have plenty of uninterrupted time, it is not important to get insurance. You should have adequate time to close.

Step 5—Close

It is best to close a few minutes before you land. That gives her the most time to get to know you, and if she says "no, thanks" to your offer of a date, less time for both of you to feel uncomfortable. If you are both going to the same city, you might ask her out for that night. That is what Phil did when he was on a business flight with some coworkers:

Last month I was flying to Seattle with two business associates. As soon as the seat belt sign went off I strolled down the aisle, checking out the women. I saw three women who appealed to me. I approached the woman at the back of the plane first and said, "Are you interested in some conversation? I get bored reading on these flights." She looked surprised and said, "Oh, no thanks. I have work to do." The two guys who were traveling with me got a good laugh when they saw that I got rejected. Then I moved on to the next candidate and said, "Would you like some conversation on the way to Seattle?" She hesitated a moment and then said, "Okay—that would be fine." When I sat down next to her, my traveling companions quit laughing. She was very good-looking.

I found out that she worked in an art gallery in New York City and would be spending one day in Seattle before going on to Alaska for an adventure travel tour. We had a leisurely conversation and got along quite well. When we were about five minutes from landing I said, "Would you like to have dinner together and see the sights in Seattle?" She agreed, saying she would be happy to have some company. Having dinner with her was a lot more fun than it would have been with the two men from work.

Phil turned his routine business travel into an adventure. His success is the result of the expertise he has developed at meeting women in that specific situation.

Tip: *When you have the flexibility in your schedule, ask your travel agent to book you on a flight that is not full. On a full flight you will have no opportunity to sit next to the woman you want to meet.*

Instead of having a boring flight, use the Five Steps to have an entertaining conversation, and possibly more, with a woman. You may not meet a woman on every flight, but you have nothing to lose by trying.

❧ 17 ❧

How to Meet a Woman While Skiing

The thrill of skiing in a beautiful mountain setting creates a light-hearted and friendly atmosphere that makes it easy to strike up conversations with other skiers. This environment is a natural for meeting women. Even though the environment is right, however, you are still not likely to wind up with a date unless you concentrate on making it happen. There is a world of difference between the success you will have if you go skiing hoping for a lucky encounter and the success you will have if you go skiing and apply the Five Steps.

The opportunities to meet women at a ski resort start the moment you step out of your car in the parking lot, because that's where you will start seeing women. There will be additional opportunities while you're in the line for lift tickets, in the lounge, and in the restaurant. The Five Steps can be used to meet a woman at any of these places. In this chapter, however, we will focus on how to meet women in three situations: waiting in a lift line, riding a chair, and skiing down a run.

Advantages of Skiing

♦ Most women who ski are in good shape.
♦ Skiing provides many unique opportunities to get near women and start conversations.

♦ With all the activity in the lift lines and on the slopes, appearing next to a woman and speaking with her will seem natural. She won't know it is a planned maneuver on your part.

♦ Because skiing is a daytime activity with an upscale clientele and a friendly atmosphere, a woman is not likely to feel threatened when you speak to her.

Disadvantages of Skiing

♦ Any given woman you approach may be involved or married. Skiing is not a singles event and, to make matters worse, ski gloves hide wedding rings.

♦ Your opportunities to meet women are limited to ski season.

♦ You may meet a woman who lives far away.

Tip: *Some ski resorts have a nationwide appeal, others attract mostly skiers from a local region. To increase your chances of meeting a woman who lives near you, ski at resorts that attract skiers from the region in which you live.*

THE FIVE STEPS WHILE SKIING

Step 1—Search

Searching can be done while you are waiting in a lift line, riding a chair lift, or skiing a run. In any of these situations, when you see an appealing woman, watch her a minute or so to see if she is with a man. This will help prevent you from approaching a woman and then having her boyfriend or husband show up.

It is easy to search while you are waiting in a lift line. Look ahead of you for appealing women in line, and watch for women getting in line behind you. It is also easy to search while riding a chair lift; simply watch the women coming down the hill as you are riding the lift up. In either of these cases, when you do see a woman you would like to meet, you usually won't be able to immediately get near her because you will be stuck in line or on the chair. In this case, "searching" really means "search and watch where she goes." You want to see where she is going (usually which run she is going down) so you can try to catch up with her. If she is behind you in the lift line, wait for her when you get off the lift and try to get near her then, or ski the run after she goes down so you can get near her when she stops to rest.

Searching for a woman while you are skiing a run does not mean sacrificing the fun of skiing. You can still have fun; just ski in a way that enables you to check out the women. Either ski fast, so you can check out those in front of you, or stop frequently to check out the women coming down the hill behind you. Ski various runs to find out which ones have the most women. In general, harder runs have fewer women. When you have completed a run and are ready to get back in the lift line, try lingering near the end of the line while you check out the women getting into line.

Step 2—Get Near

When you get in a lift line, don't immediately yell "single" (for those of you who have never ridden a chair lift, "single" is shorthand for "Is there anyone riding the chair alone?" To make the lift lines move faster, skiers try to fill the chairs to capacity). Before yelling "single," check out women near you to see if any are appealing and close enough to talk to. If so, you may choose to talk with them. Otherwise, yell "single" and give yourself a chance to meet a woman in line ahead of you.

> **Tip:** Don't get in a lift line. Instead, wait near the end of the line and watch the women getting in line. When you see an appealing woman, get in line behind her, ask if she is "single," and strike up a conversation.

Getting near a woman who is skiing down a run is not as hard as it might seem. Most skiers take occasional rest breaks when skiing a run. These rest breaks are your key to getting near a woman. Let the woman you want to meet ski a short distance in front of you. When she stops to take a break, stop near her and be ready to say something. If she doesn't take a rest break and skis to a lift line, get in line behind her (and of course ask if she is "single").

Tip: *If you are skiing with a friend, split up when you reach the lift line. Then you (and your friend if he or she is unattached) can yell "single" and have a chance to meet someone.*

Step 3—Break the Ice

Any comment on the weather, the ski conditions, or her ski outfit will make a good icebreaker. For example, you could say:

"Nice [cold, windy] day, isn't it?"

"Isn't this a great run?"

"Is that outfit as warm as it looks?"

At a ski resort, like anywhere else, what you say is not really important. But it is important that you say *something*. Someone has to start the conversation.

Step 4—Continue the Conversation

Now that you have started a conversation, your first priority is to talk with her for a while to establish rapport. Skiing is a natural subject for conversation. You could say:

"How long you been skiing?"

"Where else have you skied?"

"What's your favorite place to ski?"

"What's your favorite run?"

"Are you here just for the day?"

If, after you make two or three such remarks, she does not seem interested in talking with you, respect her wishes. Leave with a friendly "Have a nice day." If her responses are friendly and she seems interested, keep talking. Eventually weave your conversation goals into the conversation.

In many meeting situations at a ski resort, you will have only a few minutes to talk. Because of this limitation, extending your time together becomes an important goal. A suggestion to ski a run together is a natural way to extend your time with her. If you have talked with her for a couple of minutes and she seems open to your company, say, "Want to do a run together?" If you are riding a chair lift together, just before you get off the chair say, "Would you like to ski down together?" If she says yes, you now have more time with her. If she says something like, "No, I have to meet my girlfriend," don't give up. Assuming that she has been friendly, follow her refusal with, "Want to get together for drinks after skiing, or maybe we could meet for lunch next week?"

Tip: *You can make offers to extend your time together more than once with the same woman. After she accepts your offer to do a run together, and you have done a few runs, suggest taking a break together. Each time she accepts such an offer, it gives you more time with her and makes a request for a date more appropriate.*

It is almost always a good idea to get insurance early in a conversation, that is, find out her first name and enough information about her work to be able to reach her there. With this information, you have a backup. You can reach her later when she is at work in case you never get to close.

During the conversation, ask her questions to see if she meets your requirements. At a ski resort it is important to find out where she is from. You can either come right out and ask her (it is a common question at a ski resort) or lead into it by saying, "Are you here just for the day?" Local skiers often come up for one day, whereas "destination" skiers usually stay longer. If you find out that the two of you live a thousand miles apart, you might want to spend your time searching for a woman who lives closer to you.

Aaron, a student in one of our classes, has refined the art of meeting women while skiing. When he and his buddy go skiing together, they have a unique way of extending their time with the women they meet. Here is what Aaron told us:

> I've developed a very effective method for meeting women while skiing. I bring along six wineglasses wrapped in a blanket, a couple of bottles of wine, and some cheese and French bread. At the top of a lift I hide my pack in the woods near a spot with a beautiful view, and then my buddy and I search for some women we would like to get to know. Sometimes we find only one woman to join us, and sometimes a group of three or four, it doesn't matter. We always have a leisurely conversation in a romantic setting. The women are invariably impressed.

Step 5—Close

At a ski resort you won't always be able to choose the moment when you close. Say you have talked with a woman for five or ten minutes, or maybe you've even done a couple of runs with her, and she says, "I have to go ski with my girlfriends now. It's been nice talking with you." If you want to go out with her, you have little choice but to close at that moment. Don't be caught off guard. When she announces that she has to leave, be ready with a response such as, "I have enjoyed talking with you. Would you like to have dinner together tonight?" If she says she is busy, come back with, "Well, how about another night?" With that question you definitely learn whether she wants to see you again. If you do make a date, be sure to get her phone number before you separate.

When a woman doesn't force you to close by saying she is about to leave, when to close is a judgment call. In a nonsingles environment such as a ski resort, asking for a date after five or ten minutes of conversation might be too soon. On the other hand, you don't want to spend six hours with a woman, ask her out, and then learn that she has a boyfriend—that's a big waste of time. As a general rule, asking a woman at a ski resort for a date after spending an hour or so with her would probably be appropriate.

Art is an acquaintance of ours who recently got a date while skiing. Here is how he applied the Five Steps to make it happen:

I'd been skiing all morning when I noticed two women ahead of me in the lift line. One of them was very attractive. They were too far ahead to arrange sharing the triple chair, so as best I could, I kept an eye on them as I rode the lift. Toward the top of the hill I noticed they were skiing down a blue run leading to the bottom of the lift I was on. When I got off the lift, I skied fast and passed them before they got to the bottom. Then I waited.

When they got in line, I got in line behind them and said, "Do you need a third?" They did (I knew they did). I positioned myself so I ended up sitting next to the woman I liked. During the ride up the hill, I talked to the two of them, a mother and her daughter. They had been skiing together all morning. Apparently the daughter was faster than her mother, because when I asked the daughter, "Would you like to ski down together?" her mother told us to go on ahead, and seemed relieved to be able to ski at her own pace. The daughter seemed pleased to be able to have a chance to ski faster.

We skied a few runs together, talking as we rode up the chair lift. When she had to leave to meet her mother for lunch, I asked her if she would like to go out sometime. She agreed and gave me her phone number.

While you are improving your skiing skills, you can also improve your ability to meet women. Skiing and meeting women can both be exciting and rewarding.

☙Epilogue☙
Now the Fun Begins

*I*f you are like most single men, you probably haven't been having much fun meeting women, but now that you have read this book, it's time for the fun to begin. This book contains all the knowledge you will need to meet women. The fun will begin as you transform this knowledge into skill (skill is knowing what to do, and having the nerve to do it).

Dan took our class on how to meet women. Here is what he told us when we checked back with him six months later and asked him if our class had been helpful:

> Your class helped me a lot. I have been using the techniques I learned in your class, and I can tell that my ability to meet women is improving. For instance, last Saturday afternoon I decided to go to Governor's Mansion—a restaurant and bar that has a reputation as a singles gathering place. I had never been there before, so when I got there I was pretty nervous. I went in anyway, applied the Five Steps, and got the phone number of a really attractive woman.
>
> What a kick! When I walked out I was so tickled with what I had done that I was chuckling under my breath. It was such a thrill to have gone to Governor's Mansion with the specific intent of meeting a woman and getting her phone number, and to walk out an hour later with the phone number of a woman I really liked. I used to hate the long periods when I didn't

have a girlfriend, but now that I am developing this new skill, I don't think I will ever be lonely again.

It might take some months for you to transform the knowledge you have gotten from this book into the ability to meet any woman you want, but if you will just go out and try, your skill will start improving. You don't have to apply all of our techniques immediately, but at least try some of them so you start making progress. Every man who is skilled at meeting women was a novice at one time.

A NOTE ABOUT OUR COMPANION BOOK, *HOW TO MEET THE RIGHT MAN*

When we started teaching classes on how to get a date, we taught separate classes for men and women. After we combined the classes into one class for both men and women, we could see how fascinated the students were to hear the point of view of the opposite sex and to learn about the problems they were having getting dates. If you would like to gain a valuable insight into the woman's perspective on the subject of how to get a date, we recommend that you read *How to Meet the Right Man* (Birch Lane Press).

Appendix A
Forms

The Type of Woman I Want to Meet	
Category	**My Requirements**
Age	
Marital History	
Children	
Religion	
Geographic	
Smoking	
Drinking	
Drug Use	
Education	
Occupation	
Financial Status	
Character	
Type of Relationship	
Interests	
Other	

Where I Will Go

(Use Your Requirements as a Guide)
(Y = Yes, N = No, M = Maybe)

Places, Activities, & Organizations	Y	N	M
Adult enrichment classes			
Aerobics classes			
Amusement parks			
Apartment bldg. pools & rec rooms			
Art museums			
Ballroom dance clubs			
Beaches			
Bicycle group tours			
Bicycling clubs			
Bike paths			
Block parties			
Book discussion groups			
Bookstores with reading areas			
Botanical gardens			
Bowling leagues			
Bus tours			
Camping clubs			
Charities			

Places, Activities, & Organizations	Y	N	M
Charity and fund-raising events			
City parks			
City streets (busy areas)			
Civic groups			
Coffeehouses for sitting and reading			
Computer user groups			
Conservation organizations			
Country and Western dance clubs			
Country clubs			
Cross-country ski races			
Cruises			
Dance spots			
Dog owners and breeders clubs			
Dog shows			
Downtown celebrations			
Environmental groups			
Equestrian clubs			
Ethnic clubs			
Festivals (music, beer, seasonal, etc.)			
Folk dancing clubs			
Food courts			

Places, Activities, & Organizations	Y	N	M
Foreign language clubs			
Gambling casinos			
Gardening clubs			
Golf courses			
Health clubs			
Hiking			
Historical museums			
Historical societies			
Homeowners associations			
Horse races			
Ice rinks			
I.Q. clubs			
Lectures			
Libraries			
Motorcycle clubs			
Natural history museums			
Outdoor adventure tours			
Outdoor clubs			
Overweight singles clubs			
Parent organizations			
Parent/school organizations			

Places, Activities, & Organizations	Y	N	M
Parties			
Playgrounds			
Poetry reading clubs			
Political organizations			
Professional clubs of various types			
Professional singles clubs			
Public speaking clubs			
Recreation centers			
Recreational vehicle clubs			
Religious organizations			
Resorts			
Roller skating rinks			
Runs and triathalons			
Sailing clubs			
Self-help and therapy groups			
Shopping malls			
Singles bars			
Single parents clubs			
Singles support groups			
Ski clubs			
Ski resorts			

Places, Activities, & Organizations	Y	N	M
Soccer clubs			
Social mixers			
Softball teams			
Swimming clubs			
Tall clubs			
Tennis clubs			
Theater groups			
Touch football teams			
Travel clubs			
Volunteer organizations			
Widows and widowers clubs			
Zoos			
Other:			
Other:			
Other:			
Other:			
Other:			
Other:			
Other:			
Other:			
Other:			

Appendix B
Wallet Reminder Cards

The Five Steps of the Active Technique

1. Search (find someone you want to meet).
2. Get Near (near enough to speak).
3. Break the Ice (start a conversation).
4. Continue the Conversation (three goals).
5. Close (arrange to see her again).
   - Get her number.
   - Ask for a date and get her number.

My Planned Icebreakers

1. _____

2. _____

3. _____

Conversation Goals

1. Get Insurance (enough information to reach her at work).

2. Qualify (does she meet your requirements?).

3. Extend Your Time Together (suggest going somewhere else right now).

Questions or Conversation Topics to Qualify a Woman

1. _____
2. _____
3. _____
4. _____
5. _____

How to Avoid a No

Consider Her:

Safety: Suggest a daytime date (e.g., lunch, drinks after work) in a busy, well-known place. Offer to pick her up or meet her there.

Comfort: Determine if she wants a simple or elaborate date, offer the option of either.

Interests: Suggest an activity she likes (determine her interests during conversation).

How to Get Better

Plan *each step before you go out.*
Practice *in your daily life:*
1. Searching.
2. Getting Near.
3. Breaking the Ice (habitually speak to strangers regardless of romantic interest).
4. Continuing the Conversation (practice getting insurance and qualifying).

How to Meet Someone at a New Place

Use a three-phase approach over several visits:

Phase 1 – Explore: Get used to the atmosphere and plan how to do the Five Steps. Don't react negatively too quickly; give the place a chance.
Phase 2 – Experiment: Try executing the Five Steps. Evaluate your results and modify your techniques as necessary.
Phase 3 – Execute: You will have learned what works.

Meet More People in Your Daily Life

As you go about your daily tasks:
- Actively look for opportunities
- Vary when and where you go (e.g., eat at a different place or time).
- Think of icebreakers on the way.
- Develop expertise at places you frequent.

Where to Go

- Any place may have compatible people.
- Any place is better than staying at home.
- Singles places have more singles, but also more competition.
- Nonsingles places probably have fewer singles and less competition.

After an Outing, Grade Your Behavior
(preferably with a friend)

Step	Grade
1. Search.	_____
2. Get Near.	_____
3. Break the Ice.	_____
4. Continue the Conversation	_____
5. Close	_____
Five Steps Overall	

Appendix C
Ideas for a First Date

If a woman is attracted to you, what you suggest for a first date usually does not matter. She would probably accept any reasonable date you suggest. But if it is a borderline case—she may be unsure of wanting to go out with you, or maybe unsure of wanting to go out with anybody—then what you suggest can make a critical difference. If the activity you propose is appealing to her, you have a much better chance of getting an acceptance.

Here are some places and activities to give you some ideas for a first-date activity:

Afternoon teas: At an English restaurant or traditional hotel.
Antique shops: Browse for the afternoon or for an hour before dinner.
Art galleries: Wander through several and comment on what you like and don't like.
Arts and crafts shows: Relaxing, interesting, and maybe educational.
Auctions: Estates, antiques, car, horse . . . use your imagination; check the paper.
Badminton: Have a few games together; you can have fun without a great deal of skill.
Beer festivals: There are lots of new microbrews to try these days.
Bicycle rides: Ride to breakfast, or lunch; have a picnic or just a ride with conversation.
Boat rides: Rowboat, canoe, sailboat, whatever is available.

Book stores: New or used; spend a couple of hours browsing together.

Bowling: Get close with a few gutterballs.

Breakfast: Go before work or have a leisurely meal on a weekend day.

Cards: Invite her to join you for a game.

Carnival: Be a kid again; win a stuffed animal, check out the rides, and eat some cotton candy.

Caving: Spelunk together.

Classes: Take a course that is of interest to both of you; have dessert afterward.

Coffeehouses: Have a little dessert and coffee. Great for people-watching and conversation.

Concerts: In a hall or arena, in a park; classical, rock, or whatever suits you both.

Costume stores: This is a bit weird, but those who try it like it. Try a few costumes on for the fun of it. It may bring out the theatrical in you.

Country drives: Enjoy the scenery and explore a small town together.

Croquet: A nice old-fashioned game followed by some lemonade—relaxing!

Dancing: Any kind you both like (if she doesn't dance, suggest taking lessons together).

Discussion groups: Books, current events, environmental, political.

Dog shows (or cat shows): These can be fun and different.

Entertainment: Check the entertainment section of your newspaper for music, comedians, plays, performance dance.

Errands: Need to pick out a new TV? Ask her along, then have dinner together.

Ethnic dining: Ethiopian, Thai, Chinese, Korean, Japanese, Greek, Italian—pick a cuisine you both like or one neither of you has tried before.

Exercise: Pump iron, aerobicize, or jog together, then have a health drink or dinner afterward.

Explore: Visit unfamiliar areas of town, drive twenty miles to a restaurant, visit new malls.

Fairs: County fairs, state fairs, medieval fairs, and people fairs are all good for wandering and people-watching.

Fishing: If you both like it, why not? If one of you hasn't tried it, get introduced to it. If neither of you has tried it, double the fun.

Frisbee: Go to the park and throw one around for an afternoon.

Gambling: If there is a casino nearby, try it out.

Games: Scrabble, chess, or checkers by a cozy fire can be romantic.

Garage sales: Spend a Saturday morning looking for treasure.

Golf: Eighteen holes or miniature can both be fun.

Grocery stores: Try a foreign or specialty store (some serve coffee or food).

Hike: After work with a picnic dinner or on a weekend.

Hobbies: Share one of your interests by visiting a hobby store (cooking, wine making, models, pottery).

Horseback riding: Western or English can make for a memorable afternoon.

Humor: Go to a comedy club, watch a comedy channel on cable, read a humor book together.

Ice skating: If the season is right or there is an inside rink, skate together for an evening or afternoon.

In-line skating: If you don't have skates, rent some and wobble around together.

Jigsaw puzzles: Or, if you prefer, crossword puzzles; both can be nice couples activities.

Lectures: Watch the paper for listings; also outdoor equipment stores, travel agents, museums, zoos, business groups, and other places may give presentations and slide shows as well.

Libraries: Browse through the stacks; read periodicals or books.

Lunch: Take a break from work and rendezvous.

Movies: Try some you both like, or that one of you likes, or that neither of you likes.

Museums: Natural history, local, art. Try a variety; go to a special showing.

Musical entertainment: Jazz, folk, punk, classical—whatever the two of you like.

Picnic: After work or on a weekend afternoon; this can be a nice change from eating out.

Ping-Pong: If your clubhouse has a table, use it.

Play music: If one of you plays an instrument, entertain the other. If both of you play, have a duet.

Plays: Attend a show together; have coffee afterward to discuss it.

Pool: There are lots of pool halls around.

Pub crawls: Brew pubs are gaining in popularity; try the ones in your town.

Races: Dogs, horses, or cars; take your choice.

Racquetball: Does your local parks and recreation or health club have a court?

Roller skating: Most cities have roller rinks. Give it a try.

Seminars: Choose a subject that interests both of you, and you will have something to talk about.

Skiing: If the season is right.

Spectator sports: Baseball, basketball, football, hockey: high school, amateur, or professional. Something to watch while you carry on a conversation.

Tennis: There are usually public courts around if you need one.

Tour: Be a tourist in your hometown. Visit historical sites and sites of interest.

TV: Watch your favorite program together.

Walk: A simple walk in the park can be relaxing and a nice way to communicate.

Wine tastings: Sampling different kinds of wine can make it a memorable evening.

Appendix D
A Sampling of Places to Go and Things to Do

Looking through an entertainment weekly paper, a daily paper, an adult enrichment class catalog, and the yellow pages, we found a multitude of places to go and things to do. Here is what we found in each of the four sources of information:

AN ENTERTAINMENT WEEKLY

In one of the entertainment weeklies that is popular in our area we found:

Music and Concerts: 67 musical events, including a free Beethoven sonata concert at a college.

Theater: 45 theater events. One event that sounded interesting was an audience-participation improvisational comedy.

Film: 14 films at college campuses, museums, and auditoriums. Everything from movie classics to travelogues.

Sports and Recreation: 25 events. The coed volleyball game and the lectures on outdoor adventures sounded as if they would be easy places at which to socialize.

Dance Performances: 3 events.

Politics: 6 events, including a panel discussion at a university on the subject of international sanctions.

Lectures and Workshops: 57 events, including a lecture for singles sponsored by a church and a museum lecture on endangered species.

Classes and Discussion Groups: 76 events, many for singles, including a class on conversation skills, a book discussion group, and several singles support groups.

Museums: 54 listed, including a motorcycle museum.

Auditions: 4 singing and acting auditions.

Volunteers: 47 groups listed that were requesting volunteers. Examples: tutoring adults in reading, ushering at a play, and assisting the homeless and the disabled.

Galleries: 67 listed, with some onetime showings, others offering continuous exhibitions.

Kid's Stuff: 18 events and classes that give single dads a way to entertain the kids (and maybe meet a single mom).

Clubs: 125 commercial establishments, many with dance floors, offering rock, jazz, folk, country music, and jam sessions.

DAILY NEWSPAPER

In the weekend section of our paper we found the following places to go:

Concerts: 35 listed.

Theaters: 38 listed.

Children's Activities: 21 listed, including a watercolor class, story time at a library, and several events at museums.

Nature: 6 activities, several suitable for children.

Events: 28 listed, many great for socializing, including a book discussion group, a travel slide show, international folk dancing, line dancing, and an art festival.

Night Life: 51 listings, mostly singles dance spots, various kinds of musical entertainment, and several comedy clubs.

Arts: 112 public and private art galleries and exhibits of painting, photography, ceramics, and pottery.

Dances: 33 listed, many for singles, including square dancing, and ballroom, Latin, and folk dancing. The dances are sponsored by various organizations, including churches and dance studios.

Singles Events and Meetings: 37 listed, including ski trips, wind surfing outings, golf, and tennis.

ADULT ENRICHMENT CLASSES

The latest catalog listed 352 classes including:

Foreign language: 23 classes.

Travel: 8 classes on in-state, national, and international travel.

Careers, Business, and Marketing: 64 classes. Everything from running a small business to multilevel marketing.

Communication: 6 classes on public speaking and one on "the art of small talk" that might be a good place to meet a single woman.

Personal Productivity: 8 time management classes.

Computer Skills: 12 classes.

Special Events: 16 events, including seminars on making yourself feel good, sex and relationships, and how to defuse verbal conflict.

Investing: 8 classes. Everything from the basics to advanced strategies.

Real Estate: 6 classes on how to buy a home.

Home Design and Gardening: 15 classes.

Art: 19 classes.

Writing: 16 classes on writing and how to get published.

Music: 9 classes and events, including several that would be great for meeting a woman, such as opera outings, a class called "Brunch and the Symphony," and another called "Wine Tasting and Classical Music".

Acting: 8 classes.

Photography: 9 classes.

Anthropology: 4 classes.

Cooking, Beer Making, and Wine Tasting: 11 classes that would be especially good for socializing.

Social Dancing: 6 classes that are great for meeting women.

Around Town: 5 events where you go in a group to explore unique bars, cemeteries, and historical sights in the local metropolitan area. Events like these are hard to beat for meeting a woman.

Connections: 7 classes that are meant for singles, including classes on conversation skills, flirting, making impressions, places to go, and discussion groups.

Relationships: 8 classes on relationship issues. Some just for singles.

Mind Works: 15 classes, addressing hypnosis, handwriting analysis, miracles, and angels.

Yoga and Meditation: 18 classes.

Health and Massage: 14 classes on subjects such as burning fat, healing herbs, and sensual massage.

Growth: 5 classes on self-esteem and taking control of your life.

Outdoors and Sports: 16 classes that would be good for socializing, including classes on learning:

> Tennis
> Rock climbing
> Fishing
> Volleyball
> Cycling
> Kayaking
> Horsemanship
> Hiking

Golf

Snowshoeing

Yellow Pages

It is helpful to know the headings to look under. Here were some useful headings we found in our yellow pages.

Band and Orchestras: 41 listed, everything from philharmonic to Polynesian.

Bicycle Tours: 19 listed, mostly commercial tours.

Books: 278 bookstores listed.

Business and Trade Organizations: 56 listed. You might find one for your profession or industry.

Charities: 16 listed (call to see if they need volunteers).

Churches: Over 200 listed. Everything from Buddhist to Baptist. Many have singles activities and organizations.

Clubs: 122 listed. Some—such as hiking clubs, tennis clubs, tall clubs, bicycle clubs, and dating services—provide a good opportunity for meeting a woman .

Coffee Shops and Coffeehouses: 77 listed, including some in combination with bookstores. Many coffeehouses have a relaxed "sit and socialize" atmosphere, and some feature musical entertainment and poetry.

Dance Instruction: 157 studios, many catering to singles. Taking group lessons will put you in contact (literally) with many single women.

Dating Services: 43 listed. If you can afford them, they can help you meet a woman.

Gourmet Shops and Food Services: 44 specialty food shops and grocery stores, many with places where you can eat, drink coffee, and strike up conversations with the women around you.

Health Clubs: 96 listings of commercial establishments. If you know what to do, they can be great places to meet a woman.

Historic Places: 4 listed. Volunteer to work at one of these places and you could meet a lot of women in one day.

Libraries—Public: 9 listed. Spend a lazy Saturday afternoon in a library, and use the Five Steps to meet a woman who enjoys books.

Museums: 83 listed. Everything from Arabian horses to steam engines.

Professional Organizations: 35 listed.

Recreation Centers: 54 listed. Mostly city parks and recreation centers that offer inexpensive workout rooms, swimming pools, racquetball courts, golf, and various classes and instruction.

Restaurants: Hundreds listed, but only look for salad-bar and cafeteria-style restaurants where you can choose where to sit (so you can sit near a woman who is alone).

Schools—Academic—Colleges and Universities: Dozens listed, many offering evening classes for adults.

Shopping Centers and Malls: Dozens listed. Those with food courts provide especially good opportunities for meeting a woman.

Singles Organizations: 9 listed, mainly "for profit" introduction services. You might try one of these if the price is right.

Skating Rinks: 13 ice and roller rinks listed.

Social Service Organizations: 248 listed.

Swimming Pools—Public: 23 listed.

Synagogues: 17 listed. Some have singles groups.